YOUR TURN

12 Steps to Get Unstuck, Get Inspired & Get Healthy

LORI PALERMO

YOUR TURN
12 Steps to Get Unstuck, Get Inspired & Get Healthy
Copyright © 2016 by Lori A. Palermo

The content of this book is for general instruction only. Each person's physical, emotional, and spiritual condition is unique. The instruction in this book is not intended to replace or interrupt the reader's relationship with a physician or other professional. Please consult your doctor for matters pertaining to your specific health and diet.

To contact the author, visit www.workingwelltoday.com

Special thanks to the team at Promoting Natural Health, LLC.
Cover Design and Layout by Amie Olson
Illustration by Amanda Filippelli
Editing by Amanda Filippelli

ISBN-10:1-944134-05-0
ISBN-13:978-1-944134-05-1

Printed in the United States of America

Dedication

This book is dedicated to all women who have struggled with weight and confidence, who have been uncomfortable in their clothes and bodies, and who have needed support but have not known how to ask for it.

And, of course, to my mother.

Contents

Preface

There are countless diet and nutrition books on the market with more coming out every day. Television and social media are buzzing with the latest diet trends. There are loads of health and fitness magazines providing the latest tips and advice. It's all great information, and there is SO much of it! How do you know what will work for you?

How many times have you tried the latest diet and failed? Let's face it. Everybody is different. Our bodies and brains respond differently to different diets. What works for you may not work for your sister or friend, and vice versa. Maybe you had great success on a diet, then you stopped it and the weight came back, along with feelings of unhappiness and defeat. It is so frustrating! You feel like you are trying so hard.

But should eating and living a healthy lifestyle be this hard?

The answer is *no!* If you are trying to follow a super strict plan that does not fit your lifestyle, you are not going to succeed. You might tough it out and lose some weight, but how long can you sustain it? Can you really drink that shake or take those powders and supplements every day for the rest of your life?

This book is not about a specific diet, fad, or trend. This book is designed to take you on a journey of self-discovery that will help you to determine where you might be getting stuck, and to provide you with tools you can use every day to focus on your goals and live a healthier and happier life. Health is about so much more than food and exercise. It is also about adjusting your mindset and believing in yourself and your worth.

I hope you will take this opportunity to dig deep and focus on what you need to start a healthy lifestyle. You are so worth it. It's Your Turn!

Introduction

I want to take a minute and tell you about my mother. She was a beautiful woman with a huge spirit and warm heart. She was boisterous and friendly and wore bright red lipstick. She would do anything to make us kids laugh, often playing the fool just to entertain us. She had a beautiful singing voice and fostered a deep love of music in all of us. She read to us and played games with us. When we were little, we used to argue over who got to cuddle with her on the couch in the evening. Somehow, she made sure we all got equal "Mom time" and that each of us felt special and important. Mom was so many wonderful things.

She was also quiet and depressed. She was emotional and complicated and I loved her dearly. I learned so much from my mom. I learned about pride, dedication, and respect. I learned how to be empathetic and kind to people and how to be generous.

I also learned how not to be. I watched my mother's health deteriorate over the years. She was overweight and unhealthy and rarely left the house. She was uncomfortable with herself to the point that she didn't want to be photographed. Sometimes she didn't even want to be seen. She is absent from our family photos and was absent from so many events in my life.

My mom spent so much time and effort caring for everyone else, but she never spent any time or effort on herself. My siblings and I had everything we ever needed, except for a healthy and active mom. My mother died at the very young age of fifty-four. I was only twenty-four at the time and I was heartbroken. I'm still heartbroken.

Still, after her passing, she continues to teach and provide for me in a new way. Watching her health decline throughout my young adulthood, I inherently knew that her disease was preventable; that simple diet and exercise changes could have improved her health and kept her with me longer. Her early passing was a warning to me to watch over and care for my own health. Although I strive to be like her in so many ways, this is one way that I choose to be different.

My mother's life-long struggle with weight, body image, and health instilled in me the steadfast belief that proper nutrition, exercise, and holistic self-care will not only prolong life but will dramatically improve the quality of life as well. Unfortunately, it took some time for this inherent knowledge to rise to the surface of my consciousness.

In the months immediately following my mother's passing, I sought comfort in all the wrong places. Of course I sought comfort in food because that is what I had been taught my entire life. I also sought comfort in alcohol. There had never been alcohol in my house growing up, and I did not experiment much with it in my youth or as a young woman, but I was lost and it temporarily numbed the pain.

Before long, I put on twenty pounds. I was desperately saddened by the loss of my mom, but sadness was soon replaced by anger. Why did she have to die so young? Why didn't she know how to take better care of herself? Why didn't anyone who loved her see it and try to help her? Then I realized that I might be heading in the same direction. Somehow, maybe it was in honor of my mother or maybe it was in fear of following her path, I found the strength to put the brakes on my unhealthy lifestyle and start to take better care of myself. The more active I became and the healthier I ate, the more I believed in the power of healthy living.

I decided that I wanted, no, that I *needed* to help others find their way to a healthy life. I enrolled at the Institute of Integrative Nutrition, where I learned about nutrition, but more than that, I learned how many lifestyle factors come together to define our health.

Now that I have studied nutrition and health, I am more convinced than ever that my mother's early death was 100% preventable. I believe in my soul that if she had known how to seek help and had learned how to take care of herself over the years, she might still be with me today. I can't help her now, but I know I can help others.

My mission in writing this book is to motivate the reader to get started on her own unique journey to a healthier life. I want the reader to discover her worth and to learn how focusing on herself and being "selfish" about her health and wellness is the most generous gift she can give to those who love her. So many lifestyle-related diseases are avoidable if we take the time and energy to care for ourselves.

I was blessed to have my mother for twenty-four years, but twenty-four years were not enough for me. I wish I had known how to help her. I wish I hadn't been afraid to offend her. I wish she wouldn't have been too proud to ask for help.

> *If wishes were changes,*
> *there'd be no goodbyes.*
> *–Nanci Griffith*

My wish for you is that you will honor yourself and your loved ones by making a commitment to care for yourself. Invest your time and energy as you work through this book to envision and attain your healthiest, happiest life. It may be challenging, but the important things in life usually are. Don't wish for your happy, healthy life. Work for it. It's your turn.

How to Use This Book

Throughout this book you will read about various lifestyle tools to help you better care for your body and mind. We'll work together to uncover some of the roadblocks that may be in the way on your current path to health and happiness. We'll explore areas such as goal setting, stress management, self-care, and of course, nourishment and movement.

This is not a quick-fix diet book. You won't read it, magically loose twenty pounds, and then go on about your life. Reading a diet book doesn't always set you up for sustained change, or get to the heart of the issues that may be causing your long-term struggles with health and weight. You must explore your current behaviors and figure out why you do what you do in order to make lasting changes.

I urge you, however, to do more than read this book. Please use this as a tool to reflect on your own experiences and situation. Take the time to really think, dig deep, and get the full benefit from the experience. Use the space provided to make notes and write down your own feelings and revelations. This isn't a library book—scribble on it, bend the pages, and use it as a tool to explore your current state of mind and figure out where you might need some additional support.

I hope that this guide will help you to seek out support, feel empowered, and make sustainable changes so that you can be an active, positive force in your own life and in the lives of those who love you.

So, turn the page and let's work together to build your happy, healthy, confident life.

PART 1

Preparing for Change

*The secret of change is
to focus all of your energy,
not on fighting the old,
but on building the new.*

-Socrates

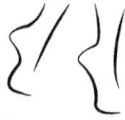

Believe in Your Worth

You must always remember...
you are braver than you believe,
stronger than you seem,
and smarter than you think.

–Christopher Robin

When we are very young, we believe that we can do or be anything. We are superheroes. We are princesses who live in beautiful castles with handsome princes. We hit the game-winning home run in game seven of the World Series. When someone asks us what we want to be when we grow up, we say that we will be football stars and race car drivers and doctors and ballerinas. There are no limits put on us. Our world is wide open.

Then, we "grow up," and through life's sometimes difficult lessons, we learn (or come to believe) that there are limitations to what we can achieve. We come to believe that we are not smart enough or pretty enough or athletic enough to be any of those things we dreamed of being. We are shaped by the world around us to believe we are not enough. We learn to be "realistic."

When we are young, we are focused solely on ourselves. Our personal well-being and our needs are all that matter. If we are lucky and grow up in a loving home, as I did, all of our needs are met. After a while, though, we learn that we should not be selfish. We learn to put others first. This is a good lesson, of course, but sometimes, we take it too far. After watching my mom work so hard to take care of us kids and always put us first, I learned that I should not focus on what I want, but rather on what others expect of me. It may not have been intentional, but my mom taught me to nobly sacrifice my own dreams and desires to do the right thing or the sensible thing or the responsible thing to please everyone else.

Granted, we all need to live in the real world. We can't fight dragons and rule kingdoms, but we need to find a balance between doing what is right and normal and expected, and doing what is right for us; that which will contribute to our happiness and well-being. We need to believe in ourselves again.

So why do we stop believing in ourselves and in our own potential? There are a lot of reasons. We are bombarded with messages from the media and from society, friends, and family about how we should be and act and look. Some of the messages are well-intended. Those who care about us want us to stay on the right path and become responsible, successful members of society. They can, however, unintentionally hold us back and shape our minds in ways that limit our potential. There are also those comments that are intended, for whatever reason, to criticize and tear us down.

When I was in high school, a classmate once referred to me as an "idealistic youth." He said it in a mean, disgusted way, like it was a bad thing. What he meant by that comment was that my optimism and positive outlook on life were not good things, but made me selfish, immature, silly, and somehow less intelligent. He was very smart and cool, so in my teenaged mind I figured he was probably right, and I took those words to heart. I tried to subdue my positive, innocent outlook in order to be "cool." To this day, I will catch myself trying to suppress my joy because I somehow feel undeserving of it.

Well, I am here to tell you that it is okay to be positive and optimistic and open to all of the wonderful possibilities life has to offer. You are not destined to stay on the path you are currently traveling. Granted, you may have more obligations and responsibilities than you had when you were a child or young adult, but you can still free your mind, pursue your dreams, and be who you are inside. It's not just okay to have a child's mind, it's absolutely essential to your happiness. Open yourself up again and consider your full potential.

Congratulations!

Congratulations! The fact that you are reading this book is proof that you believe in yourself, at least on some level, and believe that you are capable of change and worthy of the time and effort it will take to get there.

You are taking the time to walk this journey of self-discovery to help uncover what might be holding you back and keeping you from making the changes that you so desperately want to make in your life. As you read the following pages, really dig into your emotions. Look at each new experience with a beginner's mind, like a child who is open to learning new things and who believes all things are possible. It's okay if you don't have all the answers right now. You have room to learn and grow and you are worth the effort!

Now we need to build on that belief and get rid of some of the obstacles that might be in your way.

Attitude Is Everything

Are you a Debbie Downer? A Negative Nancy? Or are you (hopefully) a Positive Patty? Does your inner voice say, "I can do it! I am worth it," or, "I can't. I'm not good enough?" Your attitude can make a world of difference in your success. That little inner voice is there all of the time, giving opinions on what you should do, what you shouldn't do, and what you are capable of doing. Sometimes it is smart and keeps you safe, but sometimes it is overly cautious. The trick is to understand when your voice is keeping you on track and when it is holding you back.

Your inner voice has been with you all of your life and has been shaped by all of your experiences, successes, and failures. It can be difficult to retrain your voice to get on board with change. Your logical brain and physical body may be ready to change, but your inner voice might be saying, "Hold on. We can't do that! We've never done that before." You may not even be aware that you have a negative attitude because you are so used to hearing that voice. If you make a conscious decision to be aware of your attitude, you can change it and make it work for you.

Try to pay attention to how your inner voice reacts in different situations. When someone invites you to a party, do you think, "Yay! A chance to socialize and have fun," or, do you think, "Ugh. I don't have anything to wear. I don't have anything to talk about. This is just one more obligation." If you approach the party with a negative mindset, chances are you will have an awful time. If you go in with a positive and upbeat attitude, you will attract other positive, upbeat people and probably have a great time.

Maybe a friend has suggested that you train and run her first 5K with her. Your negative mindset says, "I can't run that far. It's too hard. I don't have time to train." Your new positive mindset will say, "That sounds like a challenge! This is a chance to have fun and accomplish this milestone with my friend. Let's go!"

Try to reframe your reactions. I hate to say, "Look on the bright side," but that is really what it boils down to. Be aware of your attitude. Be positive. Turn, "I can't do it," into, "It will be challenging for me, but I will give it my all."

YOUR TURN

Think of a recent situation in which you reacted negatively. Try to imagine how you could have put a positive spin on it.

Situation: _____

_____

_____

_____

_____

How you would normally react:_____

_____

_____

_____

_____

Reframed reaction:_____

_____

_____

_____

_____

Self-Sabotage is the Enemy

Are you your own worst enemy? Do you beat yourself up and belittle yourself? Do you take negative actions to counteract the very things that you say you want in life and then justify the negative action with excuses? Yeah. We all do it to some extent, but why? There could be any number of reasons based on your own personal situation. Here are some things to consider.

Failure is familiar and comfortable – You may be sabotaging your own success in order to remain in your comfort zone of what is familiar and feels safe. I am chronically sleep deprived, yet I often refuse to go to bed early even when I can't keep my eyes open. Why do I do this to myself? Well, it is something I am working on. I think it is because I've always operated in a sleep deprived state and I am used to it. It doesn't feel good and it's not what I want, but it is familiar.

Perhaps you are sabotaging your healthy eating or weight loss efforts because losing weight could open the door to unfamiliar situations. You may be concerned that changing your eating habits or losing weight would change your relationships with friends or with your significant other. Sometimes food and weight struggles are the very foundation of some of our relationships. You are not sure what might happen if you change, so your subconscious mind won't let you go there.

Feeling unworthy of success – You work hard at the gym, eat healthy most of the day, and then erase all of your efforts by

24

binging on cookies in the evening. Why? Perhaps you are trying to cancel out your exercise success with unhealthy eating because you don't feel like you deserve to be healthy and fit.

Attempting to stay in control – Have you ever heard of someone who breaks off a promising relationship because she is afraid of getting hurt? This is nothing more than an attempt to remain in control of the situation. You end up in exactly the same place you are afraid of being, but you control the way that it happens. Similarly, you might sabotage your weight loss in order to feel like you are in control.

Fear of failure – You don't go to the interview for your dream job because you "know" you won't get it, or you don't sign up for the 5K because you are afraid you can't complete it. Instead of taking a chance and trusting in the possibilities, you sabotage your chances of success right from the very start to avoid failure.

Playing the victim – We all know them. The lovable loser who just can't get ahead because of some other person or circumstance that is holding her back. She might say, "My mother was heavy, so I am predisposed to being overweight." Or, "I can't exercise because I hurt my knee some twenty years ago." Or, "I try so hard, but I just can't win because of x, y, or z. The universe is against me." This is the perfect way to avoid taking responsibility for your own actions and situation. Everything is someone else's fault.

What are your excuses? The first step in moving forward is taking responsibility for your own actions, or lack thereof. You are in control of your life, even though it may not seem that way sometimes. Sure, you have to be flexible and work within your family structure, time constraints, and budget, but there is room for you in there. You just need to reshape some of the beliefs that may have gotten you stuck in the practice of putting yourself last. Let's explore some of those beliefs, a.k.a. excuses!

> *"I'm too busy to focus on my health."*
> *"I have to take care of my family first."*
> *"I am not a priority."*
> *"I'm not worth the effort."*

Sound familiar? Sure. With work, family, and other obligations, it can seem like every minute of every day is taken up. This was a big issue for me for many years. I worked well beyond forty hours per week in a stressful corporate job. I also attended part-time classes to get my bachelor's degree, then my MBA, then my health coaching certificate, all while working at that job. Each time I finished with school, my time filled with other activities and obligations. It is hard to imagine how I had the time to go to school, but the reality is that I did.

Just like so many activities that you fit into every day, you can make time for yourself. The fact is that whatever needs to get done, generally does get done. You just have to schedule time for yourself as you would any other activity that is a priority.

We will discuss time management more thoroughly in the *Taking Action* section of this book. For now, I just want you to take away the idea that you DO have time and you are WORTH the time.

In case you haven't figured it out yet, YOU are a *priority* and you need to start thinking of yourself that way. If you are self-sacrificing and taking care of everyone else first, then chances are, you are not at your best. If you are not at your best, you are not giving your best to others. Ever been on an airplane? When the flight attendant goes over the safety rules, she tells the passengers to put on their own oxygen mask first in an emergency, before assisting others. You can't help others if you cannot breathe yourself. Similarly, in your life, you cannot really care for others if you don't care for yourself first.

> *"I'm too far gone to change."*
> *"I'm too old to change."*

You are not broken, maybe a little damaged and in need of some loving care, but not broken beyond repair. One of my favorite quotes is from George Elliott, who said, *"It is never too late to be what you might have been."* I take that one to heart. I even have a paper weight on my desk with that quote in it. I spent many days stuck in my corporate job, dreaming of a career where I would be able to help people get fit and healthy. Eventually, I took action and worked toward changing my circumstances.

Change is hard, but it is not impossible. You have to change your mindset and change your actions to reach your goals. It is never too late to change your career, your mind, or your health. You just need to start . . . ***Today.***

Y🌿UR TURN

Think honestly for a minute about the excuses that you tell yourself or tell others about what is holding you back. You may not even realize they are excuses because they are real to you and you believe them. Now consider how you might reframe that excuse.

For example, if your excuse is that you cannot exercise because of a bad knee, make a list of all of the other types of exercise you could do that wouldn't hurt your knee, such as swimming, possibly spinning, seated exercises with weights, etc.

When you overcome an excuse or idea that has been holding you back, you will feel motivated and free.

_____

_____

_____

_____

_____

_____

_____

_____

_____

_____

Self-Acceptance is Your Best Friend

No matter where you are and how far you have to go on your journey to a healthier life, it is so important to accept and love yourself at every step of this journey. Too often, we treat our friends and loved ones so much better than we treat ourselves. When a friend is having a bad day or is down on herself, we say something uplifting and positive to help and support her. Unfortunately, we say things to ourselves that we would never say to a friend! Start treating yourself with the same love and respect that you would give a friend.

Where you are now is where you are now, and that is okay. Stop comparing yourself to everyone else. Someone will always be thinner or smarter or richer than you. It is okay to love yourself and respect where you are knowing that you have the power to change.

There are so many negative, self-sabotaging practices we subscribe to, but I think the most damaging is negative self-talk. Comments like, "I'm fat," or, "I'm stupid," do nothing to improve your situation. Sure, you may be overweight or even obese, but please, please stop telling yourself that you are fat. Instead of thinking, "I'm fat," which is nothing more than a negative statement, consider telling yourself that you are in the process of losing weight and getting healthier, and perhaps even that you will never be this weight again. Thinking about it in that way reframes the idea of being fat, stuck, or a victim into the fact that you are working toward a better situation. It is a thought of action rather than negativity. It is a motivating statement.

Give yourself some love. Visualize where you want to be and the changes that you want to make, but think about them in a positive, action-oriented way.

_____ Y🍃UR TURN _____

Think of a negative statement you commonly make about yourself. Try to restate it in a positive, action-oriented way.

Comment: _____

_____

_____

_____

_____

Action-Oriented Statement:_____

_____

_____

_____

_____

Great!

Your head is in the right place! Your inner voice is on board. Try to keep it in check as we move through the following chapters.

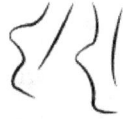

Assess Where You Are

Start where you are.
Use what you have.
Do what you can.

–Arthur Ashe

The past is over. No matter how many times you dredge it up and relive old pain or old regrets, you are not going to change anything. That's all in the rearview mirror. Your happy, healthy life is up ahead in the windshield. You have chosen to change your life now. So, start from where you are. I'm not going to say that the past doesn't matter because it does. There are reasons you got to this point and it is important to learn from them. However, you can't live there, wallow in it, and let it hold you back.

Chances are, you've tried to get healthier a few times, or a few hundred times. Maybe you've tried dozens of diets or different exercise fads. It doesn't matter how many times you have tried and failed or succeeded and slipped, or never tried at all. The most important thing is that you are here now and you are ready now. So let's start from here.

But where is here? Where are you exactly? You at least kind of know the answer to that question, but can you put it into words? "I'm overweight," or, "I'm stressed," or, "I'm unhealthy," is not your story. It goes much deeper than that. There is so much more to you than that. You need to look at the whole picture.

Now is the time to think about what is good in your life as well as what is causing you pain. You might not even be fully in touch with your true feelings. Your personal thoughts are all jumbled up in your head along with your kids' activity schedule, your grocery list, and that presentation you have to give at work tomorrow. If we are going to focus on making a positive change in your life, you need to focus on your thoughts and feelings as well. You need to really know yourself.

Now is the time to explore your inner thoughts and get them out—verbally, on paper, in a video, or whatever works for you. There are so many things I know (or think I know) in my head, but cannot articulate in a conversation because I have not really thought them through or written them down or said them out loud before. I get a better understanding of what is in my head if I force myself to verbalize it or write it down. For me, writing and journaling on the physical page is most therapeutic, but everyone is unique. Use whatever fits you.

Okay. This may feel like that time in college when you had to write a term paper but had no idea how to get it started. Luckily, you don't have to dust off the encyclopedias here or get your outline approved by your professor. This is about you. All you need to do is look inward and write what you feel. I understand that may be easier said than done, so here are some suggestions to get you started.

_____Y♥UR TURN_____

Try to answer these questions honestly and thoughtfully. The answers don't have to reflect major happenings. The smallest moments contribute to your overall mindset. Just really think before you answer.

At this moment, what is good in your life?_____

_____

_____

What are you grateful for?_____

_____

_____

What happened today that made you smile? _____

_____

_____

When was the last time you laughed until you cried? _____

_____

_____

When was the last time you cried? Why? _____

_____

_____

What causes stress in your life? _____

_____

_____

What causes you pain?_____

_____

_____

What do you like about yourself?_____

_____

_____

What would you like to change in your life?_____

_____

_____

This is the start of your story. You need to be in touch with what is good in your life as well as what you want to change before you can take action. Otherwise, you are not seeing the entire picture.

When I originally decided to write this book, the subject matter was very different. I wanted to tell the story about how I was unceremoniously downsized from a career and company to which I had dedicated twenty-eight years of my life. I wanted to tell a story about how to be resilient and adaptable to change. I wanted to tell *my* story. Most of what I wrote in the first months is not included in this book because I discovered that what I was writing was not relevant to my message or helpful to my reader. However, the process of writing my feelings and thoughts was extremely therapeutic and *so* worth the time. I was able to unclutter my mind, unload some of the negative feelings, and coach myself through what could have been a really difficult time in my life.

So, I encourage you to take the time to be honest with yourself and get in touch with your inner thoughts and feelings. Doing so will free your mind, help you find clarity, and prepare you to focus and be successful in making the changes you desire in your life. The following are two tools you can use to tell your story.

Journaling

Buy yourself a pretty notebook or journal and grab your favorite pen. You can journal on a computer if you are more comfortable, but I find there is something very personal about pen and paper. Plus, you can doodle and draw to better express your emotions. Write when you have some personal time and space (or make personal time and space).

You might want to write in the evening before bed to reflect on the day, or you might want to do it first thing in the morning to set your feelings and intentions for the day, or both. Just take fifteen minutes, or whatever time you have, to record your thoughts and feelings. Be honest, but try to keep it positive. Have a conversation with your journal and get personal.

_____YOUR TURN_____

Take fifteen minutes now and write your feelings and intentions for the rest of the day.

_____

_____

_____

_____

_____

_____

_____

_____

_____

_____

_____

_____

_____

_____

_____

_____

_____

_____

_____

_____

Free Flow Writing

Another great tool for getting your thoughts and feelings out is to just start writing your freely flowing, random thoughts. This is not the same as what you would write in your journal. You don't have to use complete sentences or really any structure at all. Your thoughts don't have to be congruent. They don't even have to make sense.

This is a sort of brain dump. Just take a few deep breaths, center yourself, and start writing whatever comes into your mind. It might go something like this, *"My feet are cold. I need to put in that load of laundry. I wonder if Julie got her new dog. It will be great to see my sister later this week. Dinner sure was good. I'm kinda full, though. We need bananas."*

You might like to do this when you first wake in the morning and are still a bit groggy. That way, you are sure not to over-think what you are writing. You might also want to do this in the evening as a brain dump before going to bed. If you get all of those random thoughts out on paper, it might keep them from banging around in your head at 2:00a.m. and keeping you awake!

YOUR TURN

YOUR TURN

Take fifteen minutes now and write your random thoughts.

_____

_____

_____

_____

_____

_____

_____

_____

_____

_____

_____

_____

_____

_____

_____

Okay. Hopefully, your head is clear and you are beginning to get in touch with yourself and your current mindset. Now let's envision where you want to go.

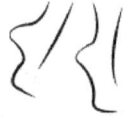

Envision Where You Are Going and Set Your Intention

The only person you are destined to become is the person you decide to be.

–Ralph Waldo Emerson

For the better part of my life I felt like I was just playing a part in someone else's life. I abandoned my creativity and my dreams to live the responsible and sensible life that was expected of me. I had a solid and successful career that had nothing to do with my values or desires as an individual. I continued my education so that I could keep climbing, climbing, climbing that ladder of success, always reaching for more, trying to do more, trying to show my value and be worthy of the responsibilities entrusted to me.

Sometimes, when I had enough energy left at the end of the

day, I would dream of doing something else, anything else. At one point, I thought I might like to be a mail carrier just so I could be out moving around instead of chained to my computer screen and tethered by my telephone headset. I was too afraid to make a change, handcuffed by money and responsibilities. Then, one day, I had an epiphany of sorts.

For years, I had been working out and trying to eat healthy, battling stress and those ten to fifteen pounds. I saw the women around me struggling with the same thing, trying to balance all of the demands in their lives while battling their own body image, self-confidence issues, and frustrations. I felt compelled to help them. I wanted to make a difference in people's lives. That's when I enrolled in nutrition school and started along the path toward becoming a health and wellness coach.

What might be surprising is that my epiphany and decision to take a new path came after my fiftieth birthday. So I can tell you that it is never too late to change direction and become the person you want to be. I guess the point is that I was the one holding myself back from doing what I wanted to do. Once I opened up and *allowed* myself to believe that change was possible, I was able to move forward.

Then synchronicity took over. With each step I took toward my desired change, God (or the universe, or whatever your chosen higher power) put the next step before me. Believe in the possibility of change and it will come.

So you see, whether you desire a career change or a stronger, healthier body, the concept is the same. Decide what you really want. Take small steps in the right direction and move forward. The universe will put the next step in front of you.

What do you envision for yourself? From time to time, in a job interview or other situation, someone may ask you where you want to be in five years. That's a great question, but I know when I was asked it, I would answer with a joke (retired and living near the beach), or with some hollow idea of where I thought I was supposed to be (the next rung up the expectation ladder). We need to dig deeper than that.

Ask your inner self: What do I really want? How do I want to feel? Can you picture what that means and how it feels at different points in time?

For Example:

General Goal: My goal is to be more active and achieve a strong, healthy body.

In 10 Days: I will feel more energized from eating a healthier diet and walking 30 minutes per day.

In 6 Months: I see myself running a 5K with my daughter.

In 1 Year: I feel confident, strong, and comfortable in my clothes.

In 5 Years: I see my healthy family and feel proud to have led my family to a healthier lifestyle by my example.

_____Y🌑UR TURN_____

Envision your goal. What does that look like in 10 days? What does that feel like in 6 months? How about a year? What about five years?

Goal:_____

_____

_____

In 10 Days:_____

_____

_____

In 6 Months:_____

_____

_____

In 1 Year:_____

_____

_____

In 5 Years:_____

_____

_____

We will talk more about goal setting in a bit. For now, I just want you to envision the change you want to see. Once you have your vision, you want to keep it in the forefront of your life. Write it down and post it on your refrigerator, on your desk at work, or wherever you will see it every day. When you read it, close your eyes for a second and envision your goal again. Feel the end result. Make it real for yourself.

You can take this a step further and create visual imagery to help you remember how you want to live and how you want to feel. You might want to create a vision board with pictures, drawings, and quotes that inspire you to keep the vision alive. Pin up a picture of an outfit that you would like to fit into, or the brochure for a race or event you would like to participate in. You could create something on a social media site like Pinterest, but I like the idea of creating a physical board that you will see every day. Get creative. If you can see, touch, and feel your goal, it will become real to you and you will never doubt that you can achieve it.

Y🌸UR TURN

Create Your Vision Board

Find some inspirational quotes that resonate with you personally and with your goal. A list of quotes I use in this book is available in the back of the book. You can start with those if you like.

Look in magazines or on Pinterest or other social media sites to find inspirational images and quotes.

Cut out pictures of happy, physically active women, or of that new dress you will buy when you reach your goal.

Handwrite and draw words and pictures of inspiration.

You now have a vision of what life will look like when you make this change and reach your goal, but maybe you are still feeling stuck. Maybe you don't believe you can achieve it. Now is a good time to think about what happens if you *don't* change. What if you do nothing? The answer is simple. If you don't take action, nothing will change. You may have heard the saying that the definition of insanity is doing the same thing over and over again and expecting a different result.

Maybe you are ready to change, but are afraid. You might not even realize you are afraid. So many times, we let our fears hold us back. To move past your fears, you need to get in touch with the reality of doing nothing. Just like you envisioned how it looks and feels to change, think about what happens if you don't change.

If I Don't Change:

In 10 Days: I will still feel sluggish and uncomfortable in my clothes.

In 6 Months: I see myself sitting on the couch while my kids play.

In 1 Year: I feel self-conscious about my weight. I am tired and unhealthy and wishing I had started a healthier lifestyle a year ago.

In 5 Years: I have just been diagnosed with a lifestyle related disease that could have been avoided if I had started my healthy diet and exercise plan 5 years ago.

Chances are, you have been thinking for some time about living a healthier and more active life. The longer you wait, the further you will have to go to achieve your goal.

Don't be afraid to fail. You can't fail if you take even one step in the right direction. Making small, sustainable changes will have a positive long-term impact on your life. Two steps forward and one little slip backward still equals movement in the right direction. You don't have to be perfect! Progress is much more important than perfection.

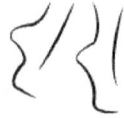

Solidify Your Goals

Setting goals is the first step in turning the invisible into the visible.

–Tony Robbins

You've now got a general picture of your new healthy life and you're excited to move forward. Let's go! Well, hold on. Let's do some more planning first. It's time to get specific about your goal. "I want to achieve a healthy body and lose weight" is a great mindset, but you are going to need a more clearly defined goal if you are going to hit the target.

One thing I learned about in my years (and years and years) in corporate America was how to set goals. At the start of each year, we would set goals against which we would measure our performance at the end of the year. It was a grueling process, and if you didn't set meaningful, measurable goals, it was difficult to make progress, and even more difficult to measure success.

So how do you set a meaningful goal?

Make it Manageable

When you are finally ready for change and full of energy and excitement to move forward, you want to do *everything* all at once. You might decide that you are going to lose fifty pounds, train for a marathon, go to the gym every day, take a vegan cooking class, and practice yoga each morning. Your list is impressive and your enthusiasm encouraged, but chances are, if you plan to do too much, you will become overwhelmed and won't accomplish any of your goals. To get started, pick one goal that you want to focus on, make some progress, and then you can add other goals as you move forward. It is important to set yourself up for success right from the beginning so that you don't get discouraged.

Also, make sure you break large goals down into manageable chunks. For example, saying you are going to lose fifty pounds can seem overwhelming. Instead, set a time frame for yourself and work backwards. You may decide you want to lose those fifty pounds in the next year, which is about four pounds per month or about one pound per week. Saying you are going to consistently lose one pound per week for the next year seems much more manageable, doesn't it? You may even decide you can lose two pounds per week, so you'll complete your goal in six months. Challenge yourself, but don't overwhelm and set yourself up for failure. Set a timeframe and choose a target that seems reasonable and doable to you.

Now, write yourself a realistic schedule and commit to it. If you decide that you will walk for thirty minutes every day at lunchtime, put it on your calendar, at least until it becomes habit for you. It may seem redundant to post it every day, but it will be much easier to stay committed if you see your plan in writing. Do the same for your yoga class or gym time. Use your electronic calendar on your mobile device if you have one. It is much more difficult to skip or "forget" your commitment to work out if a reminder pops up on your calendar.

Track your progress. You might like to keep a spreadsheet or use an app on your mobile device. Use whatever method feels right for you. I keep a small pocket calendar where I record my weight and workouts every day. This helps me to keep an eye on any trends with my weight and easily reference my workout history. The advantage of tracking your progress is that you can celebrate each little win (or loss!) and more easily recover from the small slip-ups. If you don't lose your pound this week, aim for two next week. Or, if you see a lot of empty squares on the calendar where you should have workouts recorded, it may be time to recommit to your goal. Track to stay on track!

Make it SMART

One very popular method of setting clearly defined goals is to use the **SMART** method to set goals that are **s**pecific, **mea**surable, **a**ttainable, **r**elevant, and **t**ime-bound.

Using the SMART method, "I'll try to exercise more," turns into, "I will exercise regularly by walking for at least thirty minutes every day at lunch time, taking a yoga class on Monday and Wednesday mornings, and going to the gym for an hour on Tuesday and Thursday evenings."

This is a specific goal.

It is measurable—you can track your activity to hold yourself accountable.

It is attainable—the time involved is reasonable, just a few hours per week.

It is relevant—this goal is relevant to your overall vision of getting healthy.

It is time-bound—you are setting a schedule for the activity.

Y🌀UR TURN

My Goal:_____

_____

How is it Specific?_____

_____

How is it measurable?_____

_____

Is it attainable?_____

_____

Is it relevant?_____

_____

Can it be scheduled or can you set a deadline?_____

_____

Make it Real

Now that you have set your goal and planned your schedule, go ahead and put it out there. If you make a goal and keep it as your own quiet little secret, chances are, you are not going to accomplish it. It is just too easy to fail. There are no consequences. So write it down, say it out loud, tell your best friend . . . tell everyone! Shout it from the rooftops, post it on your bathroom mirror, or put it in a frame on your desk. Consider posting your goal on social media and asking all of your online friends to hold you accountable for reaching your goal. This can be scary, but it is a great way to commit. You might also be surprised by the support you will receive or by the others you may inspire!

When you are defining and speaking about your goal, use strong words of **action**. Don't say, "I *hope* to lose fifty pounds this year," or, "I'll *try* to exercise more." Words like "hope" and "try" are not words of action. Use strong, action words like *I WILL*. "I will lose fifty pounds by the end of December by losing one pound per week," is a much stronger, more specific, and determined statement. It sounds like you actually believe you can do it, not just that you will sort of try a bit and accept failure if you don't.

Setting meaningful, well-defined goals is essential to the success of any plan. Now it's time to trust yourself and move forward.

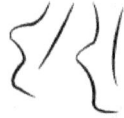

Take a Leap of Faith

Sometimes your only
available transportation
is a leap of faith.

–Margaret Shepard

We rely on faith every day whether we even think about it or not. You introduce yourself to a stranger, apply for a new job, or decide to take a cooking class. You decide to change your hair or paint the living room a new vibrant color. All of these things are little leaps of faith. The simple act of loving someone is a leap of faith. You take the leap because you believe that the person will be responsive to you, or that you will be able to complete the course, or that you will be successful in the new job. I ask you to have that same faith in your ability to care for your health and well-being. It might be difficult, but you can do this. Just have a little faith in yourself. You are certainly capable and definitely worth it.

When you have faith in yourself, you are unstoppable. Faith translates into confidence. It is about trusting your heart and your gut. It might not even be a conscious thought or decision that drives you. Sometimes you just feel that pull toward a course of action, like you know deep inside that it is time for a change. When you are true to yourself and believe in your own potential, you are living your true authentic life and anything is possible.

For many years, I was unhappy in my job. I felt trapped, like I was living someone else's life. I longed for a more fulfilling career that would make me feel useful and alive. It took me twenty-eight years, but I finally came to realize that the only thing trapping me in that job was my own fear of leaving it. Sometimes we become comfortable being uncomfortable. It is familiar. We would almost rather be miserable than risk the uncertainty of making a change. I can tell you this. Things will work out the way they are supposed to work out. That's faith. Faith means knowing that if the step beneath your foot disappears, another will appear. There will always be another step in your path to lead you to the end result. You just have to trust yourself and follow the path.

So how do you combat that self-doubt or fear when it creeps in? Fear is that point when your "logical" mind takes over and you start rationalizing all of the reasons why you can't change. That logic is manufactured in your brain and is a product of all of your rationalizations and fears and excuses. On the other hand, that tug in your gut is your heart trying to pull you in the right direction. The beauty of following your true path is that is it unwavering. If you miss a step or stumble, the path is there for you to return to. Committing to stepping onto the path is the hardest part.

You may have breezed through the goal setting and planning sections of this book, but still might feel stuck. Now is the time to take that leap into action. Give yourself permission to feel the fear and acknowledge any self-doubt. Then replace those feelings with trust and excitement. Exchange fear of the unknown with anticipation and curiosity for the potential of what might be, and relish the experience. This is exciting stuff. You are about to make a positive change in your life.

Take a deep breath. Go ahead and leap. And if you don't quite make it, leap again. Even Olympic long-jumpers get multiple attempts to perfect their leap. Trust in your abilities and remember that you don't have to make a giant leap or disruptive change in your life. Start with one little hop, and then another. You will build your confidence as you continue on your journey.

_____Y🌑UR TURN_____

Let's do a simple meditation exercise to get in touch with your strength and help you to take the leap into action.

- Sit comfortably in a chair with your feet flat on the floor, or sit cross-legged on a cushion on the floor if you prefer.

- Rest your hands, palms up, on your thighs. Sit up straight with shoulders back so that you can really fill your lungs with air.

- Close your eyes and breathe deeply in through your nose, filling your lungs and belly with air. Blow the air out of your mouth. Continue to breathe this way until you feel totally relaxed.

- Ask yourself what you really want. Concentrate on your goal. Envision yourself with that goal fulfilled. You may be picturing yourself lighter or happier.

- With each breath in, imagine you are filling yourself with confidence, strength, and energy. Perhaps you picture a color, like gold or orange.

- With each breath out, imagine you are expelling negative thoughts and fears. Perhaps you picture the exhale as gray clouds leaving you.

Continue this exercise for 10 minutes or as long as you feel comfortable. Open your eyes and feel the strength, clarity and confidence within you.

Taking Action

The most difficult thing
is the decision to act.
The rest is merely tenacity.

–Amelia Earhart

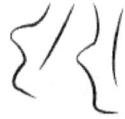

Get Support

*Refusing to ask for help
when you need it is
refusing someone the
chance to be helpful.*

–Rick Ocasek

A child does not hesitate to ask for what she needs. In fact, young children positively demand what they want. We come into this world with an innate belief that we deserve the things we desire. Why, as adults, do we feel we are less worthy and less deserving of the things we want and need? When does that notion kick in that says, "I don't need any help?" Maybe it begins when your three-year-old self begins to assert her independence and decides, "I can do it myself!" Independence and self-sufficiency are important parts of childhood development, but somewhere in adulthood, some of us cross a line.

Growing up, I was taught the importance of being smart and strong and self-sufficient, and I was fiercely proud of my independence. As a young woman, I worked hard so that I could pay my own bills and make my own way. I went to school part time, worked full time, cut my own grass, baked my own bread, and managed my own finances. Heck, I even did my own taxes! I thought I could do it all and I didn't need any help, thank you! All of the balls were in the air, but eventually, it became difficult to keep them all there. I ended up overwhelmed, overweight, overtired, and well, over it.

As women in this modern and liberated world, we are driven to believe that we can, and should, do it all. We are superwomen who perform the roles traditionally performed by men as well as those traditionally performed by women. We have stressful careers, maintain the home, have babies, cook, drive the kids everywhere, assist our aging parents, manage the finances, and perform countless other tasks every day. We are smart and strong and capable, and it is awesome. It is also exhausting!

Carving time out of your already jammed schedule for your own personal health and well-being can seem impossible. So what do you do? Which ball do you have to drop to make room for you? None of them have to be dropped. You just need to set your priorities and ask for (and accept) support.

Ask for (and Accept) Help

You are a strong, capable woman. We have already determined that. You, however, are *not* an island. You most likely have family and friends who are in your corner, ready to support you on this journey. There are a number of ways they can help, if you let them. Accepting their help will allow them to be supportive, and will give you more time to focus on your goals.

- Got a teenager who drives? Send her to run errands or pick up a few things at the grocery store. I used to love going to the store for my mom right after I got my driver's license. It gave me an excuse to drive somewhere on my own and it made me feel helpful and independent.

- Is the carpet in desperate need of vacuuming? It doesn't take a genius (or you, specifically) to do it. Ask a family member to vacuum.

- Can't leave the kids to go to the gym? Swap child care with a friend who also wants to go to the gym.

- Encourage your husband to get fit by trading off household responsibilities so that each of you gets time to go for a walk or run.

- Incorporate the family into your fitness routine. Go on family walks and hikes. Play basketball or football in the backyard. Race each other. Bike together. You'll not only get your own movement in, but you'll be teaching your family to live a more active life in the process.

Consider the possibility of hiring help as well. Yes, you are worth it. Many women pay for child care so that they can go to work. This is seen as a necessary financial trade-off for having a career. Consider other areas where it might be worth paying for support. What about house cleaning for example? Uh oh, you "do-it-all-ers" just cringed. I can relate. I grew up believing that only super rich, super spoiled women had someone else clean their house. Think about it though. Is this the best use of your time? Could you support another business by allowing them to take care of the house cleaning? Sometimes it is just more efficient to leave some tasks to the experts.

Hiring others and asking for support from family and friends are a few ways you might consider to find some additional time for yourself. Perhaps you also need to support yourself in this area. Maybe you are taking on more responsibility than you need to.

The Power of "NO"

I am a people pleaser and I am willing to bet that many of you reading this book are people pleasers as well. You want to be helpful and do what is expected of you by taking care of everyone around you. You're always doing the "right" thing and keeping those around you happy and content before worrying about your own needs or desires. That's admirable and generous. I fully support generosity and doing the right thing, but it should not be to your own detriment.

People pleasers tend to get sucked into doing all sorts of things. We manage the bake sale, host the family reunion, drive the carpool, take on the extra project at work, and on and on. Our families and bosses give us extra work to do because they know we will take it on and it will get done. Worse than that, we often volunteer for things that we don't have time for simply because no one else has volunteered and we feel an obligation to assist.

What would happen if you ever said, "No?" Would the world end? Probably not. It is pretty likely that if you said no to a request, someone else would step up and take care of it. If you say no often enough, it is also possible that people will stop asking so often. I am certainly not suggesting that we shirk our responsibilities and become selfish, isolated people. Just consider the power of, "No," once in a while so that you have more time and energy to say, "Yes," to the things that you need to do for yourself.

YOUR TURN

Think about a time when you volunteered for or agreed to do something knowing that you didn't have the time or resources to do it? How could you have responded or handled the situation by saying "No?" Remember, "No," is a complete sentence. You don't have to apologize or explain yourself.

_____

_____

_____

_____

_____

_____

_____

_____

_____

_____

_____

_____

_____

_____

_____

_____

Set Expectations

Starting any process or change in your life can be extremely difficult. It is difficult for you, the individual, to make the change, and it can be difficult for those around you to accept that you are changing. Friends and family expect certain behaviors and actions from us and that is how they define us and relate to us. When you begin to change, it can feel like a struggle because you are trying to escape or reshape the mold that you are currently in. You are shaking up the norm and that has a ripple effect on those around you.

Where Are You?

If your family is used to you being available and on the couch every evening, they may not understand the new you who wants to spend an hour in the evening walking or going to the gym. Set the expectation and explain why you need this time. Encourage them to join you or suggest other things they may do in the time when you are gone (like the dishes!).

If you engage your loved ones in your new activities and lifestyle, it will be much easier for them to get on board and support your efforts. It will also give you the opportunity to positively impact their health. When I first started running, my husband kept busy with other chores and activities while I was gone. Soon, however, my enthusiasm for running caught on and my husband decided to join me on my runs. It has turned into a great bonding experience for us. It is something that we share and it brings us closer together every time we go out for a run. Oh, and my husband's cholesterol has improved dramatically as well!

What the Heck Is on My Plate?

If your family is used to the "you" who brings cakes, cookies, and processed foods into the house, makes heavy meals, or suggests fast food for dinner, they may have a hard time accepting the new you who wants to cook lighter, healthier meals at home. Have you ever tried to serve kale or quinoa before? You might get some push back. However, healthy food can taste great.

A few years ago, I incorporated "Meatless Monday" into my weekly menu. My favorite dish on Meatless Monday became my now famous "Scrambled Grains and 'Shrooms." This is a wonderful, light, and easy-to-make dish of quinoa, mushrooms, and onions held together with a couple of beaten eggs. I also make a mean sweet potato and black bean chili, as well as mushroom lentil soup, and other great tasting healthy recipes. Even my meat-and-potatoes husband likes these healthy vegetarian dishes. You might be surprised at what your family will like. They might be surprised as well. So mix it up. If you do the meal planning in the house, you hold the power to challenge and change your family's tastes. Look for more information about food in the Nourish section of this book.

Your Eating Habits Are Annoying!

You are now more concerned about the food that you are putting into your body. You have a right to control it. I learned this lesson from my step-son who is a body builder. He has the willpower and resolve of a champion and he is not ashamed or embarrassed to manage his diet and eat the way he wants to eat regardless of what anyone else thinks about it.

I host all of the holidays and family get-togethers at my home. My husband comes from a large Italian family with very strong traditions, especially when it comes to food. When I joined the family and started hosting the holidays, I learned all of the ins-and-outs of a Palermo family dinner from my mother-in-law. Of course, we serve a lot of pasta and there is a lot of cheese, with more cheese shaken on top. I sneak in some healthy choices and skinny down recipes where I can, but I maintain the family traditions and serve the food that they want at these gatherings.

My step-son often brings his own food to these dinners. I found this extremely annoying at first. Why can't he just eat what we have?! Then, as I moved to a healthier lifestyle, I came to understand it. He wasn't going to compromise his healthy habits for the holiday, or for the family, or for my feelings, or anything. Smart kid!

I had the opportunity to exercise this food autonomy revelation last spring. I needed a little reboot to my healthy lifestyle and decided to do a ten-day low-carb, no sugar program. It just so happened to fall during my birthday and Easter. I hosted Easter and had the traditional spread for my family, but I also included some healthier options. It turned out that the family loved the new, lighter additions to the menu. When it was time to cut the cake, I just didn't take a piece. No big deal. The family structure did not come crashing down.

Food had always been such a central part of the holidays for my family growing up, and in this family that I joined. It never occurred to me that maybe the food was not the most important part of the holiday. Had I been a food pusher all of these years, contradicting my own healthy lifestyle by imposing, "Eat-this-or-you'll-hurt-my-feelings," or, "C'mon, just have a piece," attitude on everyone else? Okay, epiphany. Message received. Another lesson learned.

Your Eating Habits Are Embarrassing!

You have the right to know what is in the food you are eating. When eating out at restaurants, it is okay to ask for what you want. You can ask what's in the sauce or ask for it on the side. Again, this is a lesson learned from my step-son. He will ask for exactly what he wants at a restaurant, regardless of what is on the menu . . . and he gets it! "No dressing, grilled please, no sauce, don't bring the bread sticks. Is there butter on the vegetables?" We roll our eyes at him, and now and then, a server giggles a bit, but he always gets what he wants! Once again, it comes down to that place of not being afraid to ask for what we want and feeling worthy of receiving it. If you don't ask, you'll never get.

You're a Party Pooper

It can be very difficult to change your eating habits when you are around friends and family with whom you have bonded over food or alcohol. Meeting the girls every Thursday for margaritas is great fun, and I believe you can still enjoy a drink or two while you are living a healthy lifestyle. However, you will likely be consuming less than you may have in the past. Your friends may be annoyed when you want to stop at just one, switch to water, or forgo the chips and salsa this time. The best thing you can do is communicate openly and explain why you have changed your eating and drinking habits. Tell them how much you need their support to do so. Your true friends will support you in your efforts.

If you traditionally bond with friends over food and drinks, consider other alternatives. Maybe Thursday night margaritas can turn into Thursday night yoga followed by tea and conversation at a cozy coffee house. Or maybe drinks and bar snacks turns into a lovely dinner at that new vegan restaurant. You have the power to choose what you want to do and you have the power to positively influence your friends as well.

What does this mean for us?

Sometimes friends and family will become threatened by your new healthy lifestyle. They may resent that you are changing because they haven't yet figure out how to change themselves. They may feel that you are leaving them behind. Offer to share your journey with them and to get healthy together!

Many years back, my sister and I joined forces and attended Weight Watchers meetings together. We enjoyed the discussion and support of the group at our weekly meetings, and we were able to support each other throughout the rest of the week as well. We shared our successes and struggles and had quite a bit of fun in the process. Oh yeah, and we both lost the weight we wanted to lose!

You can also engage your friends in your exercise routine. If you need a little motivation, having a workout buddy can be a great advantage. Whether you are going to a gym, going for a run or going for a walk, chances are, you are more likely to show up if someone else is there waiting for you. Also, you may find that the time passes more quickly and your workout is more enjoyable when you have a friend to talk and laugh with. If you're a competitive person, your workout buddy can be a motivator (or antagonist) as well because you can challenge and compete against each other.

Find the Emotional Support You Need

Perhaps your friend is not interested in taking your journey with you. That's fine. Perhaps she could assist you by acting as an accountability partner. Excuse me. A what? An account-ability partner is like a confidant who gives you tough love and helps you to stay on track. You tell your accountability partner of your intentions and then ask her to follow up and hold you accountable to do what you say you will do.

For example, if you intend to walk thirty minutes every day at lunch time, you might ask your accountability partner to call you at noon and ask you if you are getting ready to head out for your walk. Don't need that much hand holding? Ask her to meet with you once a week to discuss your successes and struggles of the past week and to help you set your intentions for the following week. This is a great way for a friend to feel needed, stay involved in your journey, and support you.

Y⬤UR TURN

List some of the habits you will be changing and how your friends and family might be affected.

Think about how you will deal with their concerns and engage their support.

Now get out there and talk to them.

_____

_____

_____

_____

_____

_____

_____

_____

_____

_____

_____

_____

_____

_____

_____

Unfortunately, not everyone has a great built-in support system. Going through this exercise, you may have determined that you just don't have a strong support system within your current family and friends. That doesn't mean that you have to be alone on this journey. Seek out like-minded people. Consider joining a health and wellness community on Facebook or follow health and fitness experts on Twitter. Join a local running club, gym, or yoga studio. There are plenty of folks out there who share your passion for a healthy life and would be happy to give and receive support.

- OR -

Consider a Health Coach

You know you can do this, but you don't have to go it alone. If your family and friends are not the right support system for you, consider a professional. A professional health coach can act as an accountability partner and support you through your journey and beyond.

Your health coach is a guide or mentor who empowers you to take responsibility for your own health. She will support and guide you in implementing lifestyle and behavior changes that will contribute to the achievement of your goals.

Y🌀UR TURN

Think about your support system.

Who have you engaged?

How will they support you?

Have you reached out to a health coach?

_____

_____

_____

_____

_____

_____

_____

_____

_____

_____

_____

Hopefully your support system is now in place, but you still have a lot on your plate. You will have to effectively plan and make room in your schedule so that you have the time you need to meet your goals.

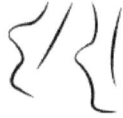

Manage Your Time

Time is the most valuable coin in your life.
You and you alone will determine
how that coin will be spent.
Be careful that you do not
let other people spend it for you.

–Carl Sandburg

Time is precious and it moves so quickly, especially when you are busy and juggling multiple priorities. How often do you look at the clock and wonder where the day went? You remember the main things you accomplished, but what happened to the rest of the time? It's time to find out.

_____Y🌱UR TURN_____

First, you'll need a notebook or calendar where you can log your time. You can get a nice purse-sized day planner at your local office supply store, or you might prefer to use a small notebook, or to create something simple on your computer or mobile device. Use whatever suits your style.

Log your time for a typical day in fifteen to thirty minute increments. This may seem like a tedious exercise, but just try it for a few days. It will be really helpful in determining where you are spending your time now and how you might adjust your schedule to fit in more time for exercise, healthy cooking, meditation, and other healthy practices going forward. This isn't a scheduling exercise. We'll get to that next. This is meant just to keep track of how you are currently spending your time. See the example in figure 1. There are no right or wrong answers. Be truthful!

Date:	Monday
6:00 a.m.	Wake-up, Make Coffee/Tea
6:30 a.m.	Have Tea, Pack Lunch, Check Emails
7:00 a.m.	Change into walking clothes
7:30 a.m.	Walked 2 miles
8:00 a.m.	Shower & Get Ready
8:30 a.m.	
9:00 a.m.	Take Kids to School
9:30 a.m.	
10:00 a.m.	Grabbed Coffee & Breakfast
10:30 a.m.	Meeting with the Tax Guy
11:00 a.m.	
11:30 a.m.	Run Errands
12:00 p.m.	Lunch & Walk with Jane
12:30 p.m	
1:00 p.m.	Work

Figure 1

Go back and analyze where your time was spent. Think about:

- How much time was spent on necessary tasks?

- Could tasks, such as errands, be organized in a more efficient way?

- How much is wasted (computer games, bad TV, reading junk email, too much social media)?

- Can anything be eliminated?

- Of the things that are important, how much of it has to be done 100% by you? Who could help with the other tasks?

Organizing Your Schedule

Now that you've got a picture of what you've been doing, let's figure out the best way to get the important things done. Do you find that you are running around scattered a lot of the time? You are crossing things off of your to-do list, but maybe not in the most efficient manner. Think about ways you can organize your tasks more efficiently to save time. If you know you have to run to the drugstore, bank, post office and grocery store today, try making a plan so that you do these things all in one outing and map them out in order. Consider grouping together other types of activities as well, like checking email only at certain times of the day, or paying the bills on the same day every week.

You can create more efficiency in your cooking as well. You are trying to cook healthier meals at home, but maybe don't have the time or energy to chop and prep and cook every night. Cooking healthy meals at home is an important part of living a healthy lifestyle. It also can take a little bit of time. However, there are cooking techniques you can employ to cook more efficiently. We'll discuss cooking quite a bit more in *Step Eleven*, but here are just a few tips related to time management.

- Get a crock pot. Spend fifteen minutes prepping in the morning and come home to a warm, home-cooked meal.

- Get the family to help with meal preparation. This will not only save you time but can be great bonding time in the kitchen as well.

- Consider doing some of your meal prep on the weekend or on an evening when you have some extra time. You could peel and chop vegetables for the week and keep them in plastic bags in the refrigerator so they are ready when needed. Sometimes the only way I ensure I'm going to have a good salad at lunch time is if I look in the fridge and find fresh veggies all ready to toss together.

- Consider preparing and freezing some meals for the week in advance. That way, if you get home late or have a rushed evening, you can pull something home-cooked and healthy out of the freezer and have dinner ready in a flash. There are some great books out there on make-ahead meals including *Make-Ahead Meal Made Healthy* by Michele Borboa, and *You Have It Made* by Ellie Krieger.

Think about other ways you can organize and budget your time in the most efficient way possible. Could you free yourself up if you reduced your social media time? Could you get up a half hour earlier? These are all personal choices and only offered as food for thought. Your schedule should be tailored to your personal lifestyle, needs, and preferences.

Y☕UR TURN

Now let's write your new schedule. Plan realistically. As you use this schedule, notice what works and what doesn't work. After you use this planning tool for a while, you get better at realistically gauging how much time things take and organizing your time in the most efficient way possible.

Date:	Monday
6:00 a.m.	
6:30 a.m.	
7:00 a.m.	
7:30 a.m.	
8:00 a.m.	
8:30 a.m.	
9:00 a.m.	
9:30 a.m.	
10:00 a.m.	
10:30 a.m.	
11:00 a.m.	
11:30 a.m.	
12:00 p.m.	
12:30 p.m	
1:00 p.m.	

Hopefully this exercise allowed you to identify some ways to better schedule your time. Chances are you discovered that all the slots are still filled with things that need to be done. You know other things will crop up and throw your schedule off. That goes without saying. So it is really important that you set your priorities.

Setting Your Priorities

We've already determined that YOU matter and that you've decided to make your health and well-being a priority, so you must make time for it. *When* you schedule certain activities can be key to making sure you get the most important things done.

I admit it. Sometimes I am a bit of a procrastinator. I may have a big project due, but I start my day reading emails and taking care of a hundred tiny things that are really not that important. When I have a deadline on a difficult project, for some reason, that seems like the perfect time to clean out my kitchen utensil drawer or take that bag of donations to Goodwill. Sometimes I avoid the important and more difficult tasks by taking care of all the little simple things first.

Also, I love to check things off my to-do list, so if there are tasks I can accomplish quickly and easily, I tend to knock those out first. The progress looks great on my list, but then as other things creep in, I find that some of the bigger, more complicated tasks don't get done because I run out of time. So how can you be sure to accomplish the important things?

You have to set your priorities. One of my favorite exercises in understanding the importance of setting priorities is the "Big Rocks" exercise. I am a very visual person, so this really helps me. It goes something like this . . .

Y⊘UR TURN

Big Rocks

- Find a large jar—this represents your available time.

- Fill the jar with a few big rocks—these represent your priorities.

- Now, put some smaller rocks into the jar—these represent other important tasks.

- Now, add some tiny pebbles into the jar—these represent other, less important tasks.

- Now, fill the jar with sand until it is full—this represents small distractions and other things that take up your time.

Everything fits if you put the big rocks in first.

- Now, dump it all out into a bucket and refill as follows:
- First, put in the sand.
- Then, the small pebbles.
- Then, the small rocks.
- Now, put the big rocks in on top.

You'll find that the big rocks no longer fit.

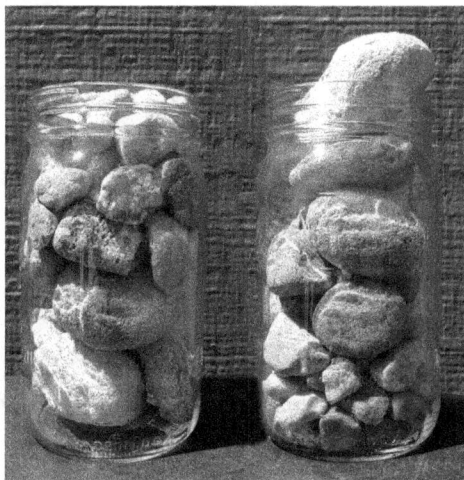

This is a visual way to understand that if you manage the small distractions and take care of the little, less important tasks first, you'll never be able to fit in your priorities. Take care of the important things first and the rest will fall into place.

Think about your priorities. What are the big rocks that have to go into the jar first? Schedule your time in such a way that the most important things get done first—work, exercise, meal planning, prepping good quality food, cooking, etc. Once that is done, take care of smaller, less important errands. Then, finally squeeze in the emails, social media, and TV time if there is any room left in your jar.

Remember: If you fail to plan, you plan to fail.

Setting priorities and creating a schedule will help you to build time into your busy life for *you*.

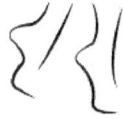

Reduce the Clutter

Keeping baggage from the past will leave no room for happiness in the future.

–Wayne L. Misner

Declutter Your Space

When I was working my corporate job, I juggled multiple priorities on a daily basis. I felt like I was moving a hundred miles per hour and running at full capacity most of the time. Constantly multitasking, it was difficult to keep everything straight. I certainly couldn't rely on my memory to keep track of everything, so I scribbled down little notes . . . everywhere. My desk was always cluttered with Post-it Notes and various scraps of paper with semi-coherent notes scribbled in barely legible handwriting. I had stacks of paper on either side of my "work area," which got smaller and more cluttered as the days passed. I called it "organized chaos" and claimed that I knew what every note meant and where everything was. The truth of the matter is that I wasted time—a lot of it—trying to find the note that I knew I wrote about the thing that was on the edge of my brain that I was trying so hard to remember. Or, I'd find a phone number with no associated name, a random date or amount at the bottom of this paper or that, and then spend time trying to figure out what it meant and if it was even still relevant. Most of this disorganized clutter didn't remind me of anything. All it did was add to my stress.

Clutter in your home can do the same thing. You know that feeling when you walk into your living room and it is strewn with newspapers, the afghan is crumpled in the corner of the couch, there's a pillow on the floor, maybe last night's popcorn bowl is still on the coffee table with some stray kernels in it. If you're like me, your chest tightens and your breathing becomes shallow. This is stress. Now, I know a messy living room isn't all *that* stressful. You can clean it up in about five minutes. The point is that even a small amount of clutter can affect your stress levels, and stress equals unhappiness, and higher levels of the hormone, cortisol, which can lead to weight gain and stress-related behaviors like overeating. So, imagine the amount of stress that cluttered basement is causing you, or how about the garage that is so full that the car has been banished to the driveway? Do we really need all of this stuff?

When my husband, Angelo, and I bought our home, his two children were living with us along with my two dogs, some fish, and a hermit crab named Leon. Over the years, the fish were flushed, the children moved out, my dear sweet dogs passed on to a better place, and I'm not quite sure whatever became of Leon. The end result, however, is my husband and I knocking around in a four bedroom house with a huge yard. I love this house and I love the yard, but we work so hard to maintain it all that we have little time for anything else. As a result, we have recently decided to downsize and move to a smaller house so that we are more agile and free. We are getting rid of much of the "stuff" in our lives and making more room for fun and experiences.

The big house had plenty of space for storage and we took advantage of that over the years. We accumulated loads of sports memorabilia, countless knick-knacks (my love of the Pillsbury Doughboy is obvious as you look around our home), and one or two of everything else. So the first order of business in our preparation to move is to begin to get rid of a lot of the stuff we have accumulated over the years. Starting this process, we pulled a few boxes out of our storage room, two of which had never been unpacked from when we moved here fourteen years ago. Hmmm. Makes me wonder how much I really needed to keep that stuff when I moved.

One of the most difficult times during the downsizing experience for me was letting go of my musical instruments and equipment. You see, at one time, I was going to be a rock star. Well, that never quite happened, but still, I hung on to this equipment for years. I guess I felt that if I gave up my instruments, I would somehow give up a piece of myself. So I called my brother who is also a musician because I knew he would understand. My brother, mind you, is not one to get rid of stuff. He's the guy who would go around on garbage day, salvaging and fixing anything that might be of use. He turned a broken clothes dryer into a compost bin, his mechanical genius saved countless lawnmowers from the scrap yard, and he has an eye for old, outdated (but really cool) amplifiers and electronic equipment. Still, I knew he would understand the pain I was feeling, so I called him. I explained that I was letting go of that part of my life and how heartbreaking it was. He told me that the guitars and amps and old cables were not what made me a musician. The musician is in me. It *is* me, and anytime I choose to bring that part of my life back, it is as simple as going to the local pawn shop with a hundred bucks and picking up someone else's past. I'm pretty sure he didn't know how profound those words were to me, but they really helped me to let go.

The musical equipment was just a start. I also have an attic full of stuff that isn't even mine. I have ancient family pictures from my grandmother's house of people who are strangers to me. I have her china that has not seen the light of day or served a meal in over thirty years. I have my mother's yearbooks from high school. If I let go of those items, does it mean I am letting go of the memory of my mother and grandmother? Certainly not! The wisdom and humor of these women lives on in my heart and one nugget or another comes to mind practically daily. They are here with me always. Their "stuff" does not have to be.

So when we let go of the stuff—the baby's old toys, the concert tickets from 1979, the old textbooks from college—we are not losing the knowledge or the memories associated with those things. We are only letting go of the physical things. Downsizing and eliminating clutter can be an arduous task, but it is freeing and can be fun. As I have sold, scrapped, and given away many of these things, I feel my burden getting lighter. Besides that, it is kind of fun to give or sell your items to someone who will actually use and enjoy them. The old guitar in the corner that does nothing but gather dust in my house will be the source of great joy for the next owner who teaches a child to play on it or uses it to entertain others. The stacks of books that I've already read will now be read and enjoyed by others. That old rowing machine will help another woman on her journey to health and wellness.

You might feel overwhelmed at the thought of reducing your clutter, but that is because the clutter is overwhelming *you*. Once it is gone, you will feel free. If you are looking for a place to start, think about your closet. You probably have clothes in three different sizes and all types of styles ranging from, "These will be back in style any day now," to, "What was I thinking?" You might even have a couple of old bridesmaid dresses stuffed in the back that you were promised *could be worn again*. All of those unused items are taking up space and increasing your stress. How many times have you stood in the midst of your overflowing closet, overwhelmed and convinced that you still don't have anything to wear? Most likely it is not that you don't *have* anything to wear. You just can't *find* anything to wear.

Anything that you haven't worn in the last year or certainly in the last two years, you most likely do not need. Donate it. Sell it on consignment. Discard it. Just get it out of your way. Make room for what is useful to you. You'll be able to see your options and make a quicker decision without feeling overwhelmed. Once your closet is clean, keep it that way. Follow the one-for-one rule. For everything coming into your closet, a similar item must go. If you buy a sweater, you must get rid of a sweater. If you buy new running shoes, donate the old pair for recycling. This keeps things from piling up.

Y🍵UR TURN

Start with one small area. Is your desk messy, or is your kitchen counter covered with mail or magazines?

- Pick one area to work on.

- Gauge how you feel when you are looking at the mess.

- Then clear the space completely, putting back only what you absolutely need, in an organized manner.

- Now, gauge how you feel looking at the clean, uncluttered space. Able to breathe now?

Remember: Your stuff does not define you. More stuff does not equal more success or happiness. However, more space and freedom does. Keep the things you use and enjoy, and get rid of the rest. Your clutter is not serving you. It is only stressing you. Work drawer-by-drawer and room-by-room to declutter your space. Clearing your space can help you gain a feeling of control over your life. That feeling can make you feel powerful and able to control other areas of your life, including your health and weight.

Make Room for the New You

Next, try clearing space in your family room, basement, or garage. You're going to want a clear, uncluttered space to work out. Clear out enough space where you can put down a mat and have some room to move. Make it attractive, a place where you'll want to go. You might use bright colors or put inspirational posters in the area. Personalize your workout space to suit your own personal style.

You are now well on your way to decluttering your physical space, but what about that space between your ears?

Declutter Your Mind

You've been there—overwhelmed, overstressed, and then everything shuts down. You can't handle another thing. You can't think. You can hardly breathe. Reducing the clutter around you can help to reduce some of that stress, but it is just as important to calm and organize your mind.

Stress is necessary for survival. When you feel stress, your body's natural "fight or flight" system kicks in. Increased adrenaline concentrates blood flow to the major systems in your body, such as your brain. The hormone, cortisol, is also released. Cortisol tells your body to stop any functions unnecessary to your immediate survival, such as digestion. The short-term effects of stress can be dizziness, headaches, indigestion, and shortness of breath. When you are in a constant state of stress, these hormones are increasing blood pressure and suppressing healthy digestion all of the time.

Chronic stress can be extremely dangerous to your health, causing issues like a weakened immune system, high blood pressure, stomach issues, anxiety, heart issues, increased blood sugar levels, and migraines to name a few. Increased cortisol levels have been linked to increased belly fat as well. Once that stress grabs hold of you, how you choose to manage it will make a world of difference in how you feel, and on your overall health.

Breathe

Breathing deeply can go a long way toward diminishing your stress. The fact is that most of us barely breathe. Studies show that the average person uses only about a third of his natural lung capacity and draws about fifteen breaths a minute (Thompson). We take short, shallow breaths from the top of our chest and ribcage area, which is known as intercostal (between the ribs) breathing, filling just the top third of the lungs. This is normal breathing for most sedentary people. When stress kicks in, your breath quickens and gets even shallower.

Counteract your stress by practicing deep breathing. Deep breathing is also known as belly breathing or diaphragmatic breathing because it engages your diaphragm. Diaphragmatic breathing is a common practice found in yoga and meditation practices. It allows you to take in more air, sends healing oxygen to your brain, improves blood flow, and releases toxins from the body, increasing energy.

Y🌱UR TURN

Measure Your Current Breathing

- Get a stopwatch or clock with a second hand.

- Breathe normally and count how many breaths you take in a minute. Chances are it is around fifteen or so.

- Now, consciously slow your breathing.

    Sit up straight, but relaxed, feet flat on the ground.

    Breathe in and try to expand your entire chest and belly, engaging your diaphragm.

    Breathe in through your nose for three counts and then out through your mouth for three counts.

    Measure your breathing for a minute now. You should now be around ten breaths per minute.

- Gauge how you are feeling. More relaxed?

YOUR TURN

Alternate Belly Breathing Exercise

- Lay on your back on the floor or on a mat, knees bent comfortably.

- Clear your mind.

- Place one hand on your belly and the other on your chest.

- When you breathe in, fill your lungs completely and expand your belly as far as possible. Feel the hand on our belly move out, while the hand on your chest remains still.

- Take thirty breaths in this manner, thinking only of your breath.

- Gauge how you are feeling.

When I was studying at the Institute for Integrative Nutrition, I was fortunate enough to attend several classes taught by Dr. Andrew Weil, a well-known expert on holistic health and integrative medicine. One of the most valuable techniques I learned for stress management is Dr. Weil's 4-7-8 breathing technique. This is my fail-safe for when stress sneaks up on me or when I am preparing to enter a situation that I know will be difficult or stressful. Although best when practiced daily, this technique is a great quick fix when you feel stress starting to take over. Give it a try.

_____YOUR TURN_____

4-7-8

- Stand comfortably or sit with your back straight and feet flat on the floor, hands in your lap, relaxed.

- Close your eyes and clear your mind.

- Place the tip of your tongue at the ridge of tissue at the top of your two front teeth.

- Blow out all the air in your lungs.

- Breathe in deeply through the nose for a count of 4.

- Hold the breath for 7 counts.

- Blow the air out of your mouth with a "whooshing" sound for 8 counts.

- Repeat 3 times.

- Open your eyes and feel the peace.

Meditation and Mindfulness

Meditation is deep breathing taken one step further. There are many different methods of meditation. Some practices focus only on the breath, while some suggest you focus on a mantra, prayer, or single word as you breathe. Some meditation practices include sounds and visualization. When you think of meditation, you may think of sitting in the lotus position on a pillow with your eyes closed, but meditation can also be done in combination with physical movement such as yoga or walking.

If you are just starting out with meditation, you might want to read more about it. There are hundreds of books on the market to choose from. I personally enjoyed reading Medication for Beginners: Techniques for Awareness, Mindfulness & Relaxation by Stephanie Clement, Ph.D. You can also take a guided meditation class online or in person, and there are countless YouTube videos on the subject. For me, meditation means walking in nature or looking out at the ocean with a clear mind and expressing gratitude for the beauty and life around me. Find the type of meditation that works for you.

Journaling

In *Step Two*, we talked about journaling as a way to get your feelings out on paper and assess your current state of being. Journaling is also a great way to clear your mind, especially using the free-flow writing technique. Hopefully, you have continued the practice of free-flow writing. If you have gotten away from it, now would be a great time to pick it up again. This is a good way to get your thoughts and feelings out and to clear the clutter from your brain. Try this first thing in the morning to get a good start on the day, and right before bed to clear your mind so that you can relax into a deep, refreshing sleep.

Expressing Gratitude

A wonderful way to reduce stress and create a more positive attitude is to practice daily gratitude. This can be part of your journaling activity or could even be part of your meditation practice.

_____Y🌿UR TURN_____

Start a Gratitude Journal

First thing in the morning, when you wake up, think about three things that you are grateful for. They don't have to be big things. You might be grateful for the warm cup of tea you are drinking, or how soft the carpet felt under your bare feet, or the fact that you woke naturally this morning without an alarm. Write these in your journal.

Pay attention to the good things that happen throughout your day. Was it gloriously sunny today? Maybe traffic wasn't too bad on the way home. Maybe you felt pretty good on your evening run. There are so many things to be grateful for! Choose at least three and write them in your journal at the end of the day.

Periodically go back and review your gratitude journal and relive the joy and appreciation.

It is also important to express gratitude to those around you. You probably say, "Thanks," quite a few times in a day without thinking much about it. Take it a step further and look the person in the eye, smile, and truly express your gratitude. Has someone done something especially nice or that helped you? Take a minute to tell them. "I really appreciated you picking up the kids today so that I could go to the gym." Or, "I'm not sure if you realize how much it meant to me when you . . .."

Finally, I know it is old fashioned, but consider writing a thank you note. I am always so touched when someone takes the time and effort to send a kind note. It makes me feel appreciated and surely does wonders for the sender's state of mind as well.

People who regularly express gratitude are 95% happier than those who do not. Okay, I made up that statistic. I don't know if that's true, but I think it has to be. If you focus on the positives in your life, you'll have little time to focus on the negatives. You might be surprised what a great life you have.

Take a Break

The superwoman in you may be offended at the suggestion of taking a break much like a tired child is offended at the idea of taking a nap. Trust me, you both need it. When you think you are too busy to take a break, chances are your work is already suffering. Sometimes even five minutes away from your stress or project can be hugely refreshing and send you back with a new attitude and a clear mind.

Take a walk around the block, do some simple stretching or breathing exercises, or even pump some light weights to get the blood flowing. Any movement will help. I keep a pair of three-pound weights next to my desk. When I need an energy boost, I do some simple arm movements with the weights to get my blood pumping. Also, walking up and down a couple flights of stairs will get you going.

Plug In

I am easily distracted. When I am trying to work or read, any other conversation, music, TV, or noise around me pulls me away from what I am doing. I simply can't concentrate. I find the distraction extremely frustrating and it stresses me out. The solution is simple, though. I can either go off on an island by myself with no distractions other than the beautiful sounds of nature (not a bad idea), or I can simulate the peaceful sounds of nature in my ears. I solved this problem for ninety-nine cents on Amazon by downloading an hour-long recording of ocean, wind and rain sounds. When the distractions around me start to stress me out, I simply plug in my earbuds and I am in my own, peaceful little world. Businesses have used this idea for years, piping "white noise" over speaker systems to bring down the level of distraction in crowded cubicle farms. I prefer my ocean sounds, thank you, but the concept is the same.

Using recorded sounds of nature is also a great way to relax or to enhance your meditation or deep breathing exercises. Sit in a comfy chair with your eyes closed, maybe burn a candle or diffuse your favorite essential oil, and take yourself to the beach, or a mountain stream, or wherever your calm, happy place may be. You can find soundtracks for free on YouTube or elsewhere on the internet, but I've found that they sometimes contain embedded advertisements that quickly jolt me out of my Zen. An hour of uninterrupted ocean sounds was worth the ninety-nine cents to me.

No Time?

There's that word again—time. Sometimes when you are super stressed, you feel like you don't have time for anything. You might think you don't have time to practice meditation or deep breathing or any other relaxation technique. Keep in mind that just five minutes of deep breathing can instantly calm you down so that you can manage whatever is stressing you out at the moment. Practicing stress-reducing techniques such as yoga, meditation, and deep breathing regularly can lower your overall stress levels and make you much more adaptable and resilient in stressful situations.

Once I started practicing regular mindfulness, meditation, gratitude, and deep breathing, I found that my overall happiness level increased. I became more calm and controlled in stressful situations. Now, when stress does start to take over, I know immediately how to manage it. Don't wait until you are stressed. Start a relaxation program today.

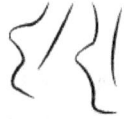

Care for You

Self-care is not selfish or self-indulgent.
We cannot nurture others from a dry well.
We need to take care of our own needs first,
then we can give from our surplus,
our abundance.

–Jennifer Louden

Care for Your Body

I can remember going to the "beauty shop" with my grand-mother. It was such a wonderful experience for a little girl. I sat in awe, watching the older women moving about, wearing pink and gray capes with curlers in their hair. Some would sit under huge dome hair dryers. All of them were talking or reading magazines. They all seemed to know each other. It was as much a social experience as it was a practical way of getting grandma's hair done. As I remember it, we would spend hours there.

Today, I dash into the place down the street for a quick haircut and I'm on my way. Somewhere along the way, I decided that spending too much time on myself was an indulgence that I didn't have time for or wasn't worthy of. So often, when we talk about caring for ourselves, we say we are pampering ourselves. The word "pamper" means to spoil, indulge, coddle, or baby. That almost sounds like you are doing something extraordinary and more than you deserve. Caring for your body and your mind is not an indulgence. It is a necessity.

There are so many ways you can care for yourself that will not just feel good, but will actually have a positive impact on your health. Read some suggestions below and choose a couple to try.

Hot Towel Scrub

Hot towel scrubbing is different from the way you may scrub in the shower or bath. It is much more of a ritual and spiritual experience than your morning shower. Here, you are standing in front of the sink, in a calm place, and giving your body some love.

Method:

- If possible, dim the lights in your bathroom.

- Light a candle.

- Run the sink full of hot water, add a few drops of lavender or other essential oil if you like.

- Soak a large washcloth in the hot water and ring out.

- Scrub your entire body, starting with the extremities and working in toward your heart. Finish with your torso and chest, ringing, and rewarming the washcloth as needed.

Benefits:

- Reduces muscle tension.

- Calms the mind and relieves stress.

- Opens pores to release stored toxins.

- Stimulates the lymphatic system to aid in the elimination of waste and toxins from your body.

- Reduces the appearance of cellulite by softening deposits of fat below the skin and allowing them to be more evenly distributed

- Promotes circulation.

Dry Brushing

Dry brushing your body has many of the same benefits as the hot towel scrub. I tend to use the hot towel scrub as a relaxation technique in the evening, but love an invigorating dry brushing before my morning shower.

Method:

- You will need a dry body brush with natural bristles. Many such brushes have a detachable long handle so that you can easily reach all areas of your body.

- Brush your entire body using a circular motion, starting with the extremities and working in toward your heart. Start at your toes and work all the way up your legs, then start at your fingers and work up to your shoulders. Finish with your torso, back, and chest.

- Don't brush too hard the first few times. Skin should be pink and energized, not red and raw. You can adjust the pressure and brush a little harder once you are used to it.

Benefits:

- Exfoliates the skin.

- Stimulates the lymphatic system to aid in the elimination of waste and toxins from your body.

- Promotes circulation.

- Reduces the appearance of cellulite.

Detox Bath

Soaking in a warm bath has long been a ritual associated with relaxation, but it is also a way to detoxify and replenish your body. First, sweating is one of your body's natural ways of eliminating toxins, so the benefits of soaking in a hot tub are obvious. Second, additives like Epsom Salt, apple cider vinegar, herbs, and essential oils have additional benefits. You can add what you like. See below for a simple detoxifying bath.

Method:

- Run a comfortably hot bath.

- Light some candles if you like or put on some relaxing music.

- Fill a large pitcher with hot water and mix in two cups of Epsom Salt, one cup of baking soda, and a few drops of lavender oil. Mixing these ingredients before pouring them into the bath will help the additives to dissolve and be better incorporated into your bathwater.

- Pour the mixture into the hot bath and mix in.

- Soak for twenty minutes, or longer if you like.

- Make sure you drink plenty of water (not wine!) during and after your bath to avoid dehydration.

Benefits:

- Detoxifies the body.

- Epsom Salt helps to replenish magnesium and eliminate toxins from the body.

- Epsom Salt also helps to reduce any muscle pain or stiffness.

- Baking soda cleans and softens the skin.

- The lavender oil has antibacterial properties, aids in relaxation, and promotes sleep.

Read the Labels on Your Beauty Products

The average woman uses a myriad of beauty products ranging from shampoos, moisturizers, makeup, and hairspray every day. I consider myself to be fairly low-maintenance, but I can think of twelve products I use almost every day in my morning routine. Did you ever stop to think about what is in those products and how they could be affecting your health?

When leading a healthy lifestyle, we pay close attention to what goes into our bodies via our mouths, but think about what might be absorbed through the skin. We know our skin will absorb nutrients. Some medications are even offered in the form of a patch and absorbed through the skin. So if medicine and nutrients can be absorbed this way, you have to think about any chemicals that you are applying to your skin.

Some chemicals in cosmetics can affect a woman's hormones, and may even cause weight gain. Read the labels on your beauty products (even though the print can be incredibly small) and research the products that you use to see if they contain phthalates, parabens, or other potentially harmful chemicals. If you want to learn more, check out safecosmetics. org or goodguide.com.

Do What Feels Good to You

There are hundreds of ways to care for your body in addition to what I've mentioned here. You could get a massage, moisturize your skin with a beautiful scent, or diffuse essential oils in your home. Not everyone will be comfortable with every method I have outlined. Find what works for you and enjoy. After all, if you aren't good to you, who will be?

Care for Your Mind

In *Step Eight*, we talked quite a bit about stress reduction techniques. There are a number of additional things you can do to care for your mind. Consider trying some of the following.

Repeat Positive Affirmations

In *Step Eight*, we discussed turning negative self-talk around to be more positive. For example, "I'm fat," turns into, "I am in the process of losing weight and getting healthier." This is a positive *I am* statement. Think about your positive attributes, your strengths. What positive *I am* statements can you list about yourself? You might say:

I am kind.

I am generous.

I am educated.

I am a good friend.

I am awesome at karaoke.

I am working toward a healthier life.

YOUR TURN

List ten positive statements describing yourself.

Refer back to this list regularly, especially when you are feeling down on yourself.

Say them out loud and believe them.

1. _____

2. _____

3. _____

4. _____

5. _____

6. _____

7. _____

8. _____

9. _____

10. _____

It is important that you know your value. No one else will appreciate you if you don't know your own worth. Happiness and positivity is a choice. When you repeat positive statements, they become the truth.

Consider the following statements. Each is a positive affirmation. Choose one or two or make up your own and say it in the mirror every day. Gear your affirmation toward goals you are trying to achieve or things that you want. Say it and believe it.

I choose happiness, success, and abundance in my life.

I am letting go of my anger and choosing to be happy.

I believe in myself and my abilities.

I am strong and deserve health and happiness.

_____YOUR TURN_____

Write down your personal positive affirmation and repeat it to yourself regularly.

_____

_____

_____

_____

_____

_____

_____

_____

_____

_____

_____

_____

_____

_____

_____

_____

_____

_____

Celebrate Your Uniqueness and Stop Comparing Yourself to Others

There is no one quite like you. No one looks exactly like you, has your smile, or thinks exactly the way you do. Your personality is a special cake baked with all of the ingredients and experiences of your life. You have your own personal little demons and your own personal joys. What makes you unique makes you beautiful and interesting.

Unfortunately, most of us spend a ridiculous amount of time comparing ourselves to others. We think, "She is more successful. She is prettier. She is skinnier," and on and on. So what? Life is not a competition. It is your own *unique* journey. You may be on a different rung of the ladder or at a different stone on the path than someone else. Heck, you might be on a different path entirely! That doesn't make you better or worse. It is just where you are now.

Try to avoid feeling animosity or jealousy towards those who appear "better" than you somehow. Those emotions do nothing to tear the other person down. All they will do is hold you back. Negative emotions are toxic to your health—mental and physical. They can cause you to give up on yourself. Celebrate that person's success and celebrate your own as well. Chances are that woman who you think has it all together is dealing with her own struggles and comparing herself negatively to yet another woman.

It is smart to pay attention and learn from others, but don't let it affect how you feel about yourself. If you look hard enough, there will always be someone who is smarter, stronger, prettier, and more successful than you are. That's okay. You are unique and wonderful. It doesn't matter if your friend has a more important job or is a smaller size than you are. Celebrate where you are now. Celebrate how far you've come. Know where you are going. It really doesn't matter if someone else gets there first.

Let Go of Anger and Resentment

You can't change the past. No amount of dreaming or wishing will change what has already happened. You can't unsay that comment. You can't undo the way you were mistreated. You can't make someone love you. You can't fix your ex. What you can do is start from where you are, make amends where they need to be made, and move forward.

We've all had disappointments in our lives. We've been in embarrassing situations. We've been hurt. The problem is when we allow ourselves to go back over it and over it in our minds and relive it until it stings all over again. The old pain, anger, or resentment does not serve you. It won't change what happened. The only thing you can change is how you choose to feel about it. Reliving the pain and anger only means it will continue to hurt you.

Life can be unfair. Someone will always hurt or disappoint you. That's not your problem. Don't let it become your prison. Learn from it, let go, and move on. The next time that old hurt starts to bubble up to the surface, close your eyes, breathe deeply, and repeat a meaningful mantra like, "I let go of my anger and pain in order to make room for joy in my life."

YOUR TURN

Releasing Your Anger

Close your eyes and visualize a red helium balloon.

Note: This exercise could be even more powerful if you are able to try it with real helium balloons.

Visualize the balloon as your anger or pain. Allow yourself to feel that pain.

What words do you associate with that feeling? Write or visualize them on the balloon.

One by one, let the balloons go and watch them float away until they are so tiny that you can't see them anymore.

Breathe deeply and feel the power and freedom that comes from letting go of that emotion.

_____

_____

_____

_____

_____

_____

_____

_____

_____

_____

Laugh, Play, Watch Cute Kitten Videos

Laughter is said to be the best medicine. We all know that laughter makes us feel good. It instantly relieves anger and tension and reduces stress. According to experts at the Mayo Clinic, there is good reason for this great feeling. "Laughter enhances your intake of oxygen-rich air, stimulates your heart, lungs and muscles, and increases the endorphins that are released by your brain" ("Stress Relief from Laughter? It's No Joke"). The effects of laughter can go beyond just making us feel good for the time being. Laughter also has long-term effects such as improving your immune system, relieving pain, and lessening depression and anxiety. Need another reason to laugh? Laughing also tightens your abs, so you might consider it somewhat of a workout.

Playing a sport or running around with your kids increases your activity level and boosts endorphins which make you happy. It can't hurt your relationship with your kids either!

And those funny cat videos online are not a total waste of your time. In a study conducted by Jessica Gall Myrick, a media researcher at Indiana University in Bloomington, participants said they felt more energetic and more positive after watching cat related online media than they had before tuning in. They also reported feeling fewer negative emotions including anxiety, annoyance, and sadness after viewing their favorite internet cats (Palermo).

The point is, take some time each day to enjoy yourself. You will lower your stress and increase your overall happiness.

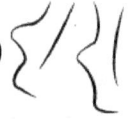

Choose to Move

*Lack of activity destroys
the good condition of every human being,
while movement and methodical
physical exercise save it and preserve it.*

–Plato

Don't Get Swallowed up by the Couch

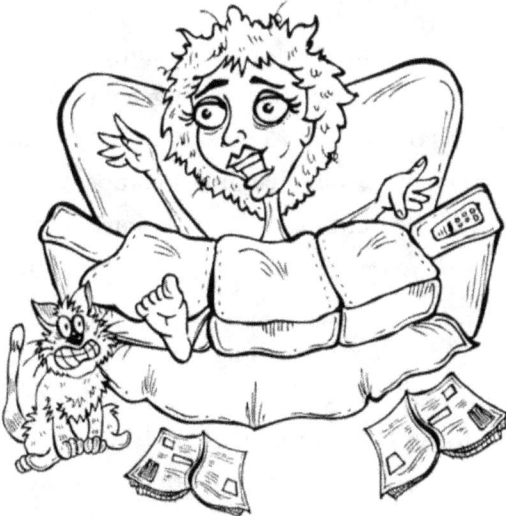

I have a friend who I've looked up to for years. I met her when I started my corporate job many long years ago. She seemed to have it all together and I was drawn to her. She was smart and put together, and she didn't seem to go in for any of the office politics or cliques. This woman taught me more than she probably realizes. She was the sole reason I went back to school to finish my degree. She practically dragged me there! She was managing school and working, and she encouraged me to do it as well. This was a big turning point for me and set me on a path of continuing education and career growth.

After twenty-some years, we were both downsized by the same company. Her position was eliminated a year before mine. Shortly after I lost my job, we met for lunch to reconnect, gossip, and commiserate. She said something during that lunch that has stuck with me. We were talking about trying to move forward after this experience because, you know, being downsized, cut, eliminated, or whatever you want to call it affects more than your employment status. It is a traumatic experience, especially after such a long tenure with a single employer. You go through a range of emotions and have to learn how to adapt to your changing situation. One thing she said to me when describing the depression and anxiety was, "You know how you just seem to get sucked into the couch?"

Yeah, I do. I think it is something that many of us feel from time to time. It is that feeling of being stuck. You just can't seem to figure out how to move ahead. Life gets difficult and we get overwhelmed and stuck. It is not because we are lazy. It is just because we can't figure out how to move forward. Hopefully, some of the self-care and stress management tips we've already discussed will help you to overcome these feelings. Still, it can be difficult to get into gear some days. You need to find your motivation. For me, it is the absolute certainty that no matter how bad or lazy or tired I am feeling before a workout, I know I will *always* feel stronger, more energized, and happier **after** the workout.

> *Remember that you will always feel better*
> *after a workout*
> *than you did before the workout.*

Certainly you might be tired or a bit sore after you exercise, but you will have a general feeling of well-being that trumps any soreness. Exercise releases endorphins—those happy chemicals in your brain that reduce pain and make you feel good all over. It also gives you a sense of accomplishment and confidence. I feel like I can tackle anything in my day after I run to the top of one particularly steep hill during my usual weekday route.

Exercise also helps to reduce depression and stress. When I'm totally stressed out and can't handle another thing, or when I'm frustrated and stuck, I know that grabbing a big glass of wine is not the answer. It's easy, but it's not the answer. I go for a run or a walk instead. Running and walking gives me clarity. It gives me time to think and allows me to release tension and stress (without the risk of a hangover). Not only will exercise release the current stress that you are feeling, but it will also make you more resilient and able to handle stress that occurs when you are not exercising.

Physical movement is good for the body, mind, and soul. Not only are you doing great things for your heart, lungs, joints, and bones when you are exercising, but you are also improving your overall sense of well-being, reducing stress, and improving your quality of sleep.

YOUR TURN

Finding Your Personal Motivation

You know that exercise is important to your health and it will make you feel great, but what really motivates you to move? What would help you get up from the couch? It might be something like . . .

- To get off of my blood pressure pills.
- To fit into that dress for the wedding.
- To be able to keep up with the kids.

Whatever it is, think about it. When the couch is sucking you in, think about your true motivation and get moving!

_____

_____

_____

_____

_____

_____

_____

_____

_____

_____

Where to Begin

You are now motivated and ready to get started. Hopefully you feel like you can do anything! And you can . . . eventually. As I've said before, it is important to start from where you are. If you have not been active for a while and jump into an intense CrossFit class or try to run three miles, you will most likely get sore or injured, become discouraged, and maybe even quit. We don't want that!

If you are new to exercise or have been away from it for a while, one of the best ways to get started is to walk. You don't need anything more than a good pair of athletic shoes and some comfortable clothes to get started. There is no set distance, speed, or duration that you must meet. Do what you can do. Depending on your fitness level, you might start with a ten-minute walk around your neighborhood. Make sure you choose a safe area and walk on the sidewalk if available, or facing oncoming traffic. Also, be visible. Wear bright clothing and carry a light if walking on cloudy days or after dark.

Each time you go out, try to go a little bit further and work your way up to at least thirty minutes of brisk walking most days. This is a great start! Now, what other activities might work for you?

What Is Your Exercise Style?

Movement and exercise are keys to good health and weight management. Any kind of movement is beneficial. You can dance, jump rope, shoot hoops, walk, run, golf, play tennis, or hang from the monkey bars. The key to sticking with an exercise program is figuring out what works for you.

It is important to fit your exercise routine to your personal style, motivation, and mood. Not everyone is a runner, or a yogi, or a weight lifter. You'll want to find something you enjoy that compliments your style and personality. There are a number of things to consider.

Personality

I admit I can be somewhat of a loner. I enjoy time alone in nature. I can walk for hours by myself just observing and listening. Walking or running alone gets me in touch with my feelings and helps me solve problems. I have made some important life decisions while walking alone. I also enjoy spinning, weight training, and yoga alone at home. It just works for me. I am accountable to myself and I know I will show up for me. Working out alone gives me clarity. As I am working my body and the blood starts flowing, my mind opens and the ideas and answers start to flow. I have no distractions and I am at peace. Body, mind and spirit—it's all connected.

If you are a bit of an introvert and a self-motivator, you may enjoy exercising alone as much as I do. You draw your energy from within and may come to enjoy your workouts as much for the alone time as you do for the physical exercise.

If you are more of a social creature, you might prefer the company of a friend or the comradery of a group when exercising. An extrovert draws her energy from others and could be motivated as much by the social aspect of the activity as the physical benefits. An extrovert may view working out alone as painful and boring. Having a workout buddy or group might also help to keep you accountable as you may be more likely to show up if you know someone else is waiting for you.

What level of motivation do you need to get moving? Do you enjoy time alone or are you more likely to work out with a buddy? Maybe you need the motivation of a professional, like a trainer. Your workout personality is definitely something to consider when developing your exercise plan.

Your personality will also affect the type of activity you choose. If you are super stressed and aggressive, you might be drawn to more aggressive activities like running or high intensity interval training (HIIT), but you could also benefit from a more calming activity, like yoga. If you are very calm and grounded, you might be drawn to yoga, but may want to try something like a Zumba class to boost your energy and break you out of your shell.

Try different things. Exercise should push you out of your comfort zone, but you should not force yourself to stick with something you absolutely hate. It just won't work. Find what you like as your fundamental go-to exercise program and then mix it up by trying new things from time to time. You always want to remain challenged and don't want to get too comfortable in your routine. As a runner, I find I get a lot of cardio and lower body work in, but I have to remember to lift weights and improve my upper body strength as well. Remember to balance yourself out.

Environment

Do you like being outside or are you more of a controlled environment kind of gal?

I will take any opportunity to go outside, so running and walking are my go-to exercises. If you like the outdoors, you might also like hiking, bicycling, roller-blading, swimming, or kayaking. The possibilities are endless, especially if you are lucky enough to live somewhere that has beautiful weather. Sometimes you might not be motivated to exercise, but the fresh air and sunshine will draw you out. Take advantage of the beautiful days and use them as motivation. Where it gets tough is when the weather is less than optimal.

When I am at home in Pittsburgh, I often have to fight rain, snow, and freezing temperatures if I am going to get outside.

I have actually come to enjoy those "bad weather" days. It is so invigorating to be outside on a chilly day when your body is warm from exercise but the chill still nips at your nose and cheeks. Running has gotten me out of the house on so many "ugly" days when I would have otherwise just cowered inside. Outside exercisers learn to enjoy all types of weather. Just make sure you are dressed appropriately and adequately protected from the elements.

If the thought of leaving your cozy heated or air conditioned space doesn't thrill you, you might consider working out at home or joining a gym.

At-home workouts can be both time and cost effective if you have the right setup. Do you have room in your home for a treadmill or workout area? You can turn the spare room or that corner of the basement into your own personal workout space with very little effort.

Depending on what activity you plan to pursue, you are going to need some room to move. Consider if there is space for the equipment you want to use—maybe a spin bike, treadmill, or rowing machine. Consider also if there is enough space to roll out an exercise mat. Is the ceiling high enough and free from overhead obstructions so that you can lift hand weights above your head, or so that you can stretch and jump? Make your workout area bright and inviting. Hang some motivational posters on the wall. Make it your happy place.

No room to work out at home? You might consider going to a gym or a studio that offers yoga, Pilates, Zumba, or other classes. Actually having to leave the house and travel to a gym or studio might be an insurmountable roadblock for someone who struggles with motivation. On the other hand, actually going someplace to workout can make you feel a sense of purpose and focus. Exercising outside of the home can give you that personal "me" time, free from distractions and interruptions. In addition, gyms and studios will have many options for classes, loads of different equipment, and perhaps even offer some coaching and training assistance.

Where you choose to work out can be an important decision. Think about your own motivations and personality. You might want to try a number of different options before you invest in equipment or purchase a gym membership.

Time of Day

When planning your workout, *when* you exercise can be just as important as where you exercise and what you choose to do. Choose a time of day that works for your schedule and is not vulnerable to getting bumped by other obligations and activities.

Are you a morning person or are you always hitting the snooze?

If you just can't seem to drag yourself out of bed in the morning, then morning workouts might not be your thing. On the other hand, I have found that working out first thing in the morning jump starts my day and energizes me for the morning ahead. Also, if you exercise first thing in the morning, your workout time is less likely to get shelved for other obligations such as getting stuck late at work or having to run the kids somewhere after school. It might be worth getting up a half hour earlier and getting it done.

If your mornings are nuts and you just can't get up any earlier, you might find you can more easily schedule your workout time for the evenings. Do what fits your schedule. Just fit it in.

Sneak Movement into Your Day

It is important to build those structured workout sessions into your day at least five or six days per week. There are so many other ways and times to squeeze some movement into your day. I call them power breaks.

At Work

One of the worst things about my former job was being chained to a desk, stuck in front of a computer, and tethered to a telephone headset. So many of us are in this situation, trapped behind a desk all day. It is not only frustrating and stressful, it is downright dangerous. You may have heard the rather frightening statement, *"Sitting is the new smoking."* According to Tom Rath, author of *Eat, Move, Sleep,* *"Sitting is the most underrated health threat of modern time. Researchers found that sitting more than six hours in a day will greatly increase your risk of an early death,"* (Nordstrom & Sturt).

Sitting for extended periods of time has been linked to a host of health issues. There is an increased risk of heart disease due to sluggish blood flow when sitting, and increased risk of diabetes due to idle muscles not responding to insulin. Too much sitting has also been linked to an increased risk in colon, breast, and endometrial cancers. Sitting also causes muscle degeneration which leads to tight hips, soft glutes, and mushy abs. It can also cause poor circulation in the legs and a foggy brain. After sitting for long periods of time, you will feel the stress on your neck and spine, especially if you are slumping in your chair. The list goes on. Even if you work out regularly, sitting all day can counteract your progress and have a negative impact on your health.

Have you stood up yet?

So what can you do if you are stuck at a desk all day? Well the good news is many employers are starting to recognize the risk and are building better workstations including adjustable desks or work counters that allow employees to stand and work. My chair in my home office is an exercise ball in a frame on wheels. Sitting on something unstable like a ball helps to engage your core muscles and legs as you sit. There is also a great option called the Swopper Chair which is like a wobbly stool that allows for vertical and horizontal movement while sitting.

There are also a number of standing desks on the market. One company makes an adjustable desktop that you can sit on any table and raise or lower throughout the day to change your position. Treadmill desks are also available so that you can actually walk while you work. I'm not sure I am coordinated enough for that, but you might like to give it a try.

If you are unable to change your desk or chair at work, you can still sneak some movement into your day. Get up and move around at least every half-hour. Put your phone on speaker and pace during conference calls. Take the long way to the restroom. Use the stairs rather than the elevator. Stretch often. Keep light hand weights under your desk and do a couple of bicep curls or shoulder presses every hour. Do partial push-ups on your desk. While sitting in your chair, lift your feet off of the floor and engage your abs. Get creative. Just take every opportunity to move.

At Home

You know you can't blame it all on the office. We do plenty of sitting at home in front of the TV as well. Train yourself to get up on every commercial break and walk around the house, do a couple of push-ups, or go up and down a flight of stairs. Better yet, turn off the TV and go outside for a brisk walk!

You can sneak movement in just about anywhere. If there are stairs, take them. Skip the drive-thru. Get out of your car and walk at every chance. If you are standing in line at the bank or grocery store, don't get annoyed. Take the opportunity to do calf raises or inconspicuously stand on one leg for eight counts, then the other. Feel yourself slumping? Straighten up and breathe deeply. Tighten your abs. Be aware of your body's inactivity and find ways to move.

Fitness Trackers

Fitness tracking devices are everywhere these days. You can monitor your sleep and your steps and just about everything else. These are great devices for keeping track of exactly how much you are moving every day. You can even find one that will buzz at you when you have been still for too long. Start with a simple, inexpensive tracker and see how you like it. I love getting feedback and tracking my activity, so my Fitbit is perfect for me. You can even compete with fellow fitness tracking friends to see who has met their goal for the day and who has a few steps left to go. The feedback can be rewarding and fun. Give it a try.

Just Do It

Okay, that's probably copyright infringement, not to mention cliché, but it's true. There are so many ways you can choose to move. You don't need to do everything at once. Just get your toes up to the starting line and get moving.

_____ Y**O**UR TURN _____

Think about your personality, schedule, and environment.

Choose what type of activity you will add to your walking routine.

Write the details: How often will you do it? Where? When?

Write this new activity into your schedule.

_____

_____

_____

_____

_____

_____

_____

_____

_____

_____

_____

_____

_____

_____

_____

_____

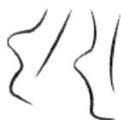

Nourish

*Our food should be our medicine
and our medicine should be our food.*

-Hippocrates

My mom was a wonderful cook and baker. I still have some of her old cookbooks including her original Betty Crocker Cookbook from 1956. It is an old three-ring binder style book. The metal spine is broken and the pages are tattered, brittle, and yellow. I don't use it anymore, but I keep it in fond remembrance of all of the wonderful meals and treats that came out of it. I also have a few recipe cards with favorite recipes written in mom's exquisite, meticulous handwriting. The cards are yellowing and splattered and stained with memories from long ago.

Yes. Mom was an amazing cook. Even with the help of her old recipes, I can't begin to recreate the magic that came out of my mother's kitchen. I can picture her to this day, standing at the counter, rolling out dough, while my sister and I hovered around or sat on the stepstool that always stood next to the counter. Mom's cooking represented warmth and happiness

147

and love. She showed us love by making delightful treats for us. Food was the center of our family celebrations. She planned and prepared magnificent family dinners, parties, and barbeques. Unfortunately, the love of food also contributed to our unhealthy lifestyle. Food was a reward for good behavior, and well, for everything. The cookie jar was always full and then quickly emptied.

Our plates were always emptied as well. We were taught not to be wasteful because Dad worked hard for our food and because there were starving children in China. Cleaning your plate was a big deal at our house. So even in my adult life, I have a hard time leaving food on my plate. This is a really difficult habit for me to break. I will catch myself from time to time eating something that I don't want so that I don't "waste" it. When you think about it, eating something your body doesn't need is more wasteful (and waist-full) than throwing it in the trash.

Mindful Eating

When do you stop eating? When the cookie jar is empty or the plate is clean? Do you sometimes not even know you are full until you are completely stuffed? You are not alone. Everything is fast these days. We drive fast, we talk fast, and we eat ... really fast. It takes fifteen to twenty minutes for your body to signal your brain that you are full and that you should stop eating. If you are eating too quickly and mindlessly shoveling food into your mouth, you can blow way past satiety before you become aware of it, causing you to eat more than you want or need. You end up stuffed, groggy, and feeling like you have a food hangover.

The other day I was super busy. I was multitasking like we all do and working on a project when I realized it was after noon and I was hungry. So I went to the kitchen to toss together my usual salad for lunch. While I was doing that, I started to peel and chop some of the veggies I'd need to make dinner. Then my phone pinged to alert me that I had a text message. I responded to the text, finished chopping my veggies, and sat down to my salad. I had my iPad in front of me and was catching up on email while I ate. I was shoveling salad and reading and thinking about my afternoon to-do list when, all of a sudden, a spinach leaf headed down the wrong pipe and I started choking. I think the choking was the only thing that brought me back to the fact that I was actually eating! I looked down at my bowl. The salad was nearly gone and I hardly remembered eating it.

Rushing through your meals is horrible for your digestion. Chewing is the first step in the digestion process as the enzymes in your saliva break down your food. Swallowing food whole and eating too quickly can cause acid reflux and other issues. In addition, if you are eating too quickly, you are most likely gulping air, which can lead to belching and stomach discomfort. Beyond that, rushing through meals can leave you unsatisfied because you do not actually enjoy your meal. Slow down and pay attention to your food. The first step in healthy eating is mindful eating.

Mindful eating starts before your meal begins. Slow down and try these tips at your next meal.

Y🌱UR TURN

Mindful Eating

- Use a plate.

- Sit down at a table . . . without your electronics.

- Before you eat, take a minute to breathe. Say a prayer or express gratitude in your own way, or just take a couple of deep breaths to slow yourself down.

- Look at your food and notice the colors and aromas.

- Try to take small bites.

- Chew and taste your food! So often, we just inhale and swallow. Some experts say that you should chew each mouthful fifty times. That can be pretty difficult to do, but try it once. You might be surprised how little you are actually chewing.

- Pay attention to the flavors and the feel of the food.

- Try putting your fork down between bites.

- Finish with a deep, relaxing breath.

- Notice your level of satiety.

When you are finished eating, it can be helpful to send yourself a signal that the meal is over. No, I don't mean with a big fattening desert. Try herbal tea. Ending your meal with a cup of unsweetened herbal tea that contains ginger or mint will not only signal the end of your meal, but the herbs and spices will also help aid digestion. You might also try a small sugar-free mint, or if possible, brush your teeth. I promise you won't want seconds if your mouth feels minty clean.

How you eat can be as important as what you eat, but we also need to understand why we eat.

Why Are You Eating?

You may notice that this step is titled *Nourish* rather than *Nutrition*. In this book, I am not going to tell you exactly what to eat or talk too much about the science of food. That would make this another diet book. I am more interested in helping you to think about *why* you are eating and why you are making the choices you are making. There is most likely some underlying reason you want that cookie or salty snack. Are you hungry or are you thirsty, sad, stressed, tired, bored, lonely, frustrated, or angry? It is important to assess your level of hunger and your state of mind to determine why you are eating. This is the first step in figuring out how to overcome bad habits and gain control of your eating.

The best way to assess your feelings and reasons for eating is to capture them in a journal. Write up your own or copy the following example. The important thing is to capture how you are feeling when you are planning to eat, and how you feel about your choice afterwards. I have also built in a couple of techniques to stall and calm yourself before deciding to eat (drink a glass of water, breathe, etc.). You can add whatever works for you, just make sure you add a block for each time you eat during the day. In the example journal, I have also provided a space where you can write your affirmation or goals in the morning so that you can be reminded of them each time you decide to eat. You might also want to conclude each day with a brief summary of your thoughts and feeling for the day.

FOOD/FEELINGS JOURNAL

Date:_____   Weight:_____

Morning Affirmation

Time:	What are you doing?	How do you feel?	Level of Hunger (1 low - 5 starving)

❑ Drink a glass of water   ❑ Take 3 deep breaths in and out

What did you eat?	How do you feel about your choice?

Time:	What are you doing?	How do you feel?	Level of Hunger (1 low - 5 starving)

❑ Drink a glass of water   ❑ Take 3 deep breaths in and out

What did you eat?	How do you feel about your choice?

Time:	What are you doing?	How do you feel?	Level of Hunger (1 low - 5 starving)

❑ Drink a glass of water   ❑ Take 3 deep breaths in and out

What did you eat?	How do you feel about your choice?

YOUR TURN

Food/Feelings Journal

- Fill out your journal every time you are planning to eat.

- Practice the techniques to stall before eating.

- Record what you ate and how you felt about it after.

- Review your journal periodically and look for patterns.

Filling out this journal honestly and completely should help you to figure out why you are eating, and help you to keep from eating when you are not truly hungry. If you find you are eating for emotional reasons, you can take action to address the root cause of your craving before spiraling down into a bag of chips. This kind of inner discovery can be difficult. Hang in there and keep working on it. I am rooting for you.

Breaking Down Cravings

Once you have used the food-feeling journal for a couple of days, you will probably begin to notice patterns to your eating. You might see, for example, that every time you ate a sweet snack, it was linked to an emotion rather than to hunger.

Emotional Eating

Emotional eating can be a slippery slope. If you give in to emotional eating, chances are it will backfire and you will feel the emotion even stronger after you have eaten. Eating will have the exact opposite effect of what you intended. Let's say you have polished off a half bag of Oreos because you were sad, lonely, or depressed. They tasted like relief going down, but now that you have eaten the Oreos, you feel sick and disgusted with yourself, which makes you even sadder and more depressed.

What can you do to break this cycle? You must try to counteract the emotion with a solution other than food. This won't be easy, but you have got to give it a try.

Are you stressed? Before you reach for the cookie, try some of the deep breathing exercises we practiced earlier. Control your stress and you control your eating.

Are you bored? Maybe zoned out in front of the TV? Don't distract yourself with a bag of chips. Get up and walk, call a friend, or keep your hands busy with an activity, like knitting.

Are you angry? Punch a pillow. Jump up and down or shadow-box to get your aggression out. Channel that negative energy into something positive, like a quick workout.

Are you lonely? That cookie is not your friend. Call a real friend or consider joining a community or group where you can engage and interact more with others.

Emotional eaters use food as a distraction from what is really bothering them. Dig deep and get to the root of what you are feeling. Then deal with that emotion in a constructive (and non-caloric) way.

Addicted Eating

This is a process of honest self-discovery. You've got to really know yourself to understand why you are eating. I know, for example, that I am a recovering sugar addict. No matter how disciplined I think I am, no cookie or piece of candy is safe if left alone with me. I simply can't have it in the house. I was raised on sugar and sweets and they are wonderful! When I was young and poor and working at my first full-time job, I ate Reese's pieces for lunch almost every day. They were cheap and right there in the vending machine, and I loved them so.

It's not totally my fault. The jury is still out on whether or not sugar is addictive in the same way as cocaine or other drugs. However, scientists do know that sugar lights up some of the same reward centers of the brain as addictive substances (Rettner). We know that it makes us happy, temporarily, and then it makes us crash.

Entire books have been written on sugar "addiction" and how to overcome it. For me, I know that I have to avoid it. If I start the day with sugar in my tea, I will crave sugar all day. If I eat one cookie, I will most likely eat six. So I am trying to retrain my taste buds to lessen the sugary hold on them. I stopped adding sugar or any sweetener to my tea and I have come to enjoy the clean, real taste of the tea. Sometimes eating sweet vegetables such as carrots and bell peppers gives me enough sweetness to overcome the desire for "junk" sugar. If you are a sugar addict like me, you have to find what works for you.

Your Body Needs Balance

What else could your cravings be telling you? Cravings aren't all in your head. A craving could be your body's way of telling you that it needs something. My step-daughter was a vegetarian for a couple of years when, all of the sudden, one day she absolutely had to have a steak. She couldn't explain why, but the craving was real and she ate the steak. A couple of weeks later, she found out that she was pregnant. The craving was her body's way of telling her that it needed iron and additional nutrients for the baby.

Your body is always seeking balance. Sometimes you think you are hungry when you are simply dehydrated. As suggested in the food-feelings journal exercise, try drinking a glass of water when you have a craving. The craving may disappear.

Your body could be craving other nutrients as well. If you are craving sugar and caffeine, it may be your body's way of telling you that it needs healthy fuel, such as complex carbs. If you have a sugar craving, don't go for the cookie. Try eating a piece of fruit instead.

Craving ice cream? Maybe your body is just overheated. Try an ice cold glass of water first.

Don't feel deprived when you turn down junk food. Feel empowered that you made a healthy choice. Unhealthy food is not a reward; it is a punishment.

The body is an amazing organism. Pay attention to it and feed it well.

When Do You Eat?

As you analyze your food-feelings journal, also pay attention to *when* you eat. Do you skip breakfast, eat lightly throughout the day, and then hit the vending machine at 3:00p.m. or devour everything in sight in the evening? If you are going to avoid cravings and feel energized, it is important to keep your body fueled and your blood sugar at even keel throughout the entire day.

The average person most likely eats smaller meals for breakfast and lunch and then consumes a much larger meal at dinner time. Consider reversing that idea. If you eat a larger breakfast, you will be fueling yourself up for the morning with sustained energy until lunchtime. Then, eat a healthy and satisfying lunch followed by a small, healthy snack in the afternoon—perhaps some carrots and hummus or an apple with peanut butter. This will keep you fueled and less likely to go crazy at dinner. Finally, end with a light dinner.

> *Breakfast like a king,*
> *Lunch like a prince,*
> *Dinner like a pauper.*
> *-Adelle Davis*

Eating this way can provide you with energy when you need it most and gives your body time to burn off calories before going to sleep.

Your Diet and Why It Matters

More than one-third of U.S. adults are obese (BMI of 30 or above). Obesity rates are even higher (39.5%) among middle-aged adults. Obesity is killing us with preventable conditions such as heart disease, stroke, type 2 diabetes, and certain types of cancer ("Overweight & Obesity: Adult Obesity Facts"). What is really sad is that our children are also becoming obese and dying of these diseases as well. We simply must set a better example and reverse this trend.

Y🖐UR TURN

Calculate Your BMI

You can find numerous BMI calculators online, but you can perform this calculation on your own as well.

- Calculate your height in inches and square that result. So if you are 5 feet, 5 inches tall, that's 65 inches squared (65 x 65) = 4225.

- Now, divide that number into your weight in pounds, so if you weigh 169 pounds, that is .04.

- Multiple that result by 703, so .04 x 703 = a BMI of 28.12.

A BMI between 18.5 and 24.9 is considered healthy, 25-29.9 is considered overweight, and 30 and up is considered obese. Keep in mind, this is not a perfect calculation, as someone with very high muscle mass may have a higher BMI and still not be overweight.

_____

_____

_____

_____

_____

_____

_____

_____

Don't worry about the BMI number. It does not define you. It is simply a reference point so that you can estimate if you are in a healthy weight range.

While obesity has numerous causes including a sedentary lifestyle, the number one cause of obesity is our diet, and the Standard American Diet (SAD) is a mess. SAD, appropriately named, has all of the factors that contribute to preventable chronic disease. It is high in animal fats, high in saturated fats, low in fiber, high in processed foods, low in complex carbohydrates, and low in plant-based foods.

We're fat, but we're fighting. There are thousands of different dietary theories out there as a testament to our desire to overcome SAD and the obesity epidemic. I recently searched for "diet books" on Amazon and I got 201,694 results. There are high-protein diets, vegetarian diets, gluten-free diets, low fat, high fat, South Beach, Atkins, paleo, and numerous iterations of each. I even found the Peanut Butter Diet and the Chocolate Diet. It is no wonder people are confused about what to eat.

Don't get me wrong. Many of these are sound nutritional plans that work for a lot of people. I just personally don't like the word *"diet."* Diets don't work. Diets end and old habits resume. Diets cause guilt, stress, and shame. Diets are about deprivation. You don't want to be deprived. You want to be **nourished.** You want to enjoy nutritionally sound, quality food. Think about how you feel when you say, "I'm on a diet." That phrase is usually accompanied by a frown and a shoulder shrug. Think instead, "I am eating healthfully!" It is a much more positive statement.

It is important to keep a positive tone when talking about your eating plan. Don't say or think, *"I can't have that."* This is a restrictive and negative statement that will probably make you feel deprived and want that food even more. Consider instead saying, *"I don't want that."* This puts you in control. You are making a choice to not eat the doughnut or the cookie. It reinforces your position that you want to eat healthy, quality foods.

What is Quality Food?

If you walk down the "health food" section of the grocery store, you will find isles and isles of processed protein bars, granola bars, shakes, powders, and supplements. Some of these items can be a good addition to your diet, depending on your personal lifestyle and metabolism. They can also be a great alternative when you need to grab something quick. You have to be careful, though, as many of the bars in this isle are nothing more than glorified candy bars loaded with sugar, chemicals, and other processed ingredients.

When you are starting a healthy eating plan, you want to nourish your body with real whole food rather than processed ingredients and chemicals. The closer you can get to real whole food, the better. Take carrots, for example. A fresh carrot contains, well, carrot. A bag of baby carrots contains carrots that have been peeled, tumbled, and sometimes processed through a bath containing chlorine. Canned baby carrots contain carrots, water, sugar, salt, and calcium chloride. Finally, consider frozen honey glazed carrots in sauce. These contain carrots, water, sugar, enzyme modified butter, dried honey, wheat starch, brown sugar, salt, modified corn starch, xanthan gum, and artificial color (ewwww!). The further you get away from the fresh carrot, the more additives and the fewer nutrients you have.

A general rule of thumb is to eat fresh whole foods when possible. When choosing processed foods, go for the shortest list of ingredients possible and watch out for added sugar, salt, and chemicals.

Should I Eat Organic?

These days, with factory farming practices, you can't even always trust your whole carrot. "Some fruits and vegetables can have nine different pesticides in a single serving," according to Jane Houlihan, the senior vice president for research at the Environmental Working Group (Evans & Leamy). Well the FDA has determined these pesticides are safe, right? According to Toxics Action Center, "Pesticides have been linked to a wide range of human health hazards, ranging from short-term impacts such as headaches and nausea to chronic impacts like cancer, reproductive harm, and endocrine disruption," ("The Problem with Pesticides").

So should you shell out the extra money for organic produce? In some cases, the answer is *yes*. Organic fruits and vegetables are grown under strict guidelines that limit the use of pesticides. Depending on growing practices, thickness of skins, etc. some produce absorbs more pesticides than others. These are considered the "dirty dozen" of the produce world. They include peaches, apples, cherries, strawberries, grapes, summer squash, spinach, kale, bell peppers, celery, and cucumbers. Where possible, it is best to buy organic when buying these fruits and vegetables. Produce less likely to be contaminated, also known as the "clean fifteen," include asparagus, avocados, cabbage, cantaloupe, sweet corn, eggplant, grapefruit, kiwi, mangos, mushrooms, onions, papaya, pineapples, frozen sweet peas, and sweet potatoes.

Did you know that the PLU code on your produce will tell you if the item is organic or not? A five-digit PLU code that starts with 9 means that the item is organic. A PLU code that starts with 3 or 4 means the produce is conventionally grown.

How can you get the freshest, most natural fruits and vegetables? Buy in season and local where possible. Shop your local farmer's market and talk to your farmer. You can ask if his products are organic and what types of chemicals are used in the growing process. Another great alternative is to join a Community Supported Agriculture group, or CSA. In a CSA, your local farmer offers a certain number of "shares" to the public. When you buy a share or membership, you receive a box or bag of the farmer's seasonal products at set times, usually weekly, throughout the growing season. To find a CSA in your area, go to www.localharvest.org/csa.

Eat in color. Adding many colorful fruits and vegetables to your diet can have a great impact on your health. Fruits and vegetables "contain antioxidants like carotenoids and antho-cyanins that give produce its color and may play a role in preventing age-related diseases like cancer and heart disease," explains Elizabeth J. Johnson, Ph.D., associate professor at Tufts University (Roberts). Try different fruits and vegetables, even if you think you don't like them. You can retrain your taste buds to enjoy healthy, fresh food if you give it a try. I never liked tomatoes until I grew my own and discovered what a real, fresh tomato tastes like.

Protein

Fruits and vegetables are extremely important to your healthy eating plan. However, you should be eating quality protein at every meal as well. You can get healthy amounts of proteins in some grains like quinoa, and also from beans, peas, seeds and nuts, such as almonds. Avocado, broccoli, and edamame are also great sources of protein. If you are not opposed to consuming animal products, you might look to eggs and dairy products such as yogurt and cottage cheese as great sources of protein. If you eat meat, poultry and seafood, make sure you eat the highest quality available. Look for fresh-caught seafood and meat or poultry that is free from additional steroids and antibiotics. Consider grass-fed beef which tends to be higher in healthy omega-3 fats and lower in saturated fat.

Grains/Carbs

You hear it all the time that carbs are bad and should be avoided. That is mostly because the Standard American Diet includes the wrong kind of carbs—simple carbohydrates such as those found in processed bread, sugary cereals, cookies, and crackers. These types of carbs spike your blood sugar quickly and then leave you feeling sluggish and tired—the typical sugar crash. The energy from simple carbs is stored as glycogen that quickly gets converted to fat if not used immediately. Simple carb foods are also generally low in nutrients.

Complex carbs, however, are a different story. Foods such as whole grain breads, bran cereals, leafy green vegetables, fresh fruits, and brown rice contain complex carbohydrates. These carbohydrates are absorbed more slowly into your blood stream and provide for more even and prolonged energy. The slow absorption can help to control appetite and delay hunger. These foods are generally high in fiber and nutrients as well.

Always look for whole grains. For example, don't buy "wheat bread" and assume it is whole grain. Look for "whole wheat" as the first ingredient on the label. Even better, look for whole grains such as brown rice, buckwheat, or whole oats.

Fats

Remember the low-fat craze? I bought into it a while back as many of you probably did. We were buying fat-free cheese, fat-free crackers, fat-free hot dogs, and just about anything else that claimed to be fat-free, thinking it was healthy. Those were the days when we were told that fat makes you fat. Sounds reasonable, but these days, more evidence points to the fact that simple carbs and sugar make you fat. Many fat-free products actually add sugar to improve taste and compensate for the missing fat. The result, unfortunately, is that in most cases, the fat-free or low-fat version of your favorite food can be worse for your health and waistline than the full-fat version.

Dietary fat is not the enemy. In fact, fat is a vital macronutrient that the body needs to function. Dietary fat supplies essential fatty acids for growth, healthy skin, vitamin absorption, and brain function. New research clearly shows that individuals eating healthy fats actually have a substantially lower *risk* for dementia (Perlmutter).

Still, there are good fats and bad fats.

Trans-Fats – These are the worst fats and should be avoided. Although now eliminated from most of the products we buy, you may still find trans fats in highly processed foods, margarine, chips, cookies, pastries, and some peanut butters. Trans fats raise bad cholesterol (LDL) and lower good cholesterol (HDL) which leads to an increased risk for heart disease.

Saturated Fats – These are the fats found in beef, poultry, pork, dairy, and palm oil. Opinions are mixed, but too much saturated fat can potentially increase your risk for heart disease.

Monounsaturated Fats – These are the fats found in avocados, olives, olive oil, nuts, sunflower oil, seeds, and some fish. These fats raise good cholesterol and lower bad cholesterol and can be considered part of your healthy diet.

Polyunsaturated Fats – These the fats found in salmon, sardines, fresh tuna, flax seed oil, walnuts, and soybean oil. They are considered to be an important part of your heart-healthy diet.

Sugar and Sweeteners

People in the U.S. consume twenty-two teaspoons of sugar per day, while the U.S. Dietary Guidelines recommend six teaspoons for women and nine for men ("Cut Back, Way Back, On Sugar, Says Heart Group"). Refined white sugar has relatively no nutrients and contributes to weight gain, bloating, fatigue, migraines, obesity, cavities, cardiovascular disease, and a host of other ailments. It can also disrupt absorption of nutrients, possibly leading to osteoporosis and depression.

Does that mean that you should switch to a sugar substitute such as aspartame, saccharin, or sucralose? Certainly not! There is no good reason to add these artificial processed chemicals to your diet. Even some so-called natural sweeteners, such as Stevia-based sweeteners, are highly processed.

If you must have something sweet, opt for a natural sweetener that provides additional nutrients. Raw natural honey, for example, provides a concentrated dose of antioxidants and has even been shown to lower cholesterol. Or try Blackstrap molasses which contains iron, vitamin B6, magnesium, calcium, and more antioxidants than any other natural sweetener. Another sweet option is 100% pure maple syrup which is rich in antioxidants and protects against inflammation.

It can be difficult to break the sweetening habit, but it can be done. The trick is to train your taste buds so that you don't need to add as much sweetness. I overcame adding sweetener to my tea and found that my cravings for sweets in general somewhat diminished. I don't miss the sweetener in my hot or iced tea anymore. I never even think about using it now.

If you still need a little sweetness in your life, try getting it from whole fruits and sweet vegetables such as bell peppers or sweet potatoes that provide additional nutrients and fiber.

Salt

Sodium is a mineral that is essential for life. It helps control the body's fluid balance. When there is extra sodium in your bloodstream, however, it pulls water into your blood vessels and increases your blood pressure. High blood pressure is the leading risk factor for women's death in the U.S. The American Heart Association recommends that people eat no more than 1,500 milligrams of sodium per day, but the average American eats more than 3,400 milligrams per day ("Sodium and Your Health").

Even if you are not addicted to the salt shaker, as I admit I was, you may still be taking in much more sodium than you realize. Processed foods contain a shocking amount of sodium. Just one cup of canned chicken noodle soup has nearly 700 milligrams of sodium. Two tablespoons of ranch dressing contain about 260 milligrams. One tablespoon of ketchup has 160 milligrams. A single-serving pouch of tuna packs 340 milligrams. Restaurant foods are even scarier. A "lighter fare" chicken dish at a well-known chain restaurant has only 590 calories, but packs a whopping 2,480 milligrams of sodium. Nutritional information for many restaurants is available online. If you know you will be eating out, check the online menu and decide what to eat before you get there. Better yet, cook at home where you can control what goes into your meal.

Try substituting different spices to add flavor rather than adding salt to your meal. Spices have many great properties in addition to enhancing the taste of your food. Many have heart healthy benefits, antibacterial, and antiviral properties, antioxidants, and trace amounts of vitamins and minerals. Spice it up, but shake off the salt!

How Much Should I Eat?

I am not a fan of counting calories. It is difficult and time consuming. We do, however, have to pay attention to portions and balance. One way to think about balancing your diet is by looking at your dinner plate. At a typical meal, half of your plate should contain fruits and vegetables, heavy on the vegetables. One quarter of your plate should contain protein (lean meat, poultry, fish, beans, nuts, and seeds). One quarter of your plate should contain whole grains such as brown rice. You should also add a tablespoon or two of healthy fats such as avocado or olive oil to your meal.

Measuring portion sizes can be difficult and our perception has gotten distorted over the years as portion sizes continue to grow. Here are some visual guidelines to help you measure your portion sizes without a scale.

1 cup, such as a serving of vegetables or fruit, is the size of your fist

3 ounces of meat, fish, or poultry is the size of a deck of cards

3 ounce grilled/baked fish fillet is the size of your checkbook

4 ounce piece of fruit is about the size of a baseball

1 ounce of cheese is about the size of 2 dice

1 teaspoon is about the size of your fingerprint

1 tablespoon is about the size of your thumbprint

Concentrate on balance and the quality of your food. If you fill up your plate with nutrient dense, fiber rich, colorful vegetables, quality protein, whole grains, and eat mindfully, you will find you are satisfied with less food.

Healthy Snacks

We've talked about cravings and how your mood affects your hunger. Let's face it, sometimes you are actually hungry between meals and need to feed your body a healthy snack. Always be prepared for these times. If you don't have a healthy snack on hand, you will most certainly hit the vending machine, drive-thru, or candy bowl. Make sure you've always got portion-sized bags of almonds, a piece of fruit, or a high quality whole food snack bar in your purse, car, and desk. At home, make sure you always have cut up vegetables and hummus sitting at the front of your refrigerator. You are more likely to reach for healthy snacks if they are readily available to you.

Hydrate

As discussed earlier, dehydration can often appear as hunger. Your body is 70% water and you need to keep it replenished and happy. Plain water is a great way to go, but there are other options as well.

Water with lemon is a great choice. It aids digestion, reduces inflammation, helps to flush out toxins, has antioxidants that improve the appearance of your skin, and has vitamin C and potassium. You can get creative and add other herbs like mint or vegetables like cucumber to your water to alter the taste and provide additional nutrients. Drinking naturally flavored water can reduce your desire to drink soda.

Green tea is another of my favorites. I drink it iced or hot and always add lemon to it as well. Green tea is low on caffeine and contains antioxidants that flush toxins from the body.

While fruit juice has many vitamins in it, juice is not necessarily a great option to drink often as it contains so much concentrated sugar. Be careful with sports drinks for the same reason, and please, put down the soda. A single twelve ounce can of soda contains sixteen teaspoons of sugar and has no nutritional value. Diet soda, I'm inclined to believe, is worse still due to its artificial sweeteners and chemicals.

Be careful with alcohol as well. Moderate drinking (One twelve-ounce beer or five-ounce glass of wine per day) is said to be good for the heart and circulatory system, and possibly protects against type 2 diabetes and gallstones. Heavy drinking, on the other hand, can damage the liver and heart. If you are trying to lose weight, you probably don't need the empty calories, but if you are going to drink alcohol, opt for red wine. Red wine contains resveratrol, an antioxidant said to guard against a variety of diseases including cancer, heart disease, and Alzheimer's disease.

Planning Your Meals

If you plan or prepare the meals in your household, you have all the power. You hold your health and the health of your family in your hands. You have the opportunity to serve fresh, nutrient rich meals or processed, sugary, and salt laden foods. It is up to you to introduce healthier foods into your diet. It might take some time to acquire a taste for the healthier version of dinner, but you can change your tastes and learn to love healthy foods.

If you still don't think you like some vegetables or are worried that your family will reject the broccoli or kale, consider the stealth method of adding vegetables to your meal. Finely chop carrots, mushrooms, and zucchini and add them to your meatloaf, casseroles, or sauces. Try using a spiralizer or julienne tool to make vegetable "noodles" and use in place of, or mixed in with, traditional noodles. Try serving spaghetti squash in place of traditional spaghetti. Add extra herbs and spices to your meals. There so many ways to healthy-up your meals and so many great recipes out there. Experiment and find what you like.

The key to serving healthy, nutritious meals is to have a plan and to do some advanced preparation. You cannot come home hungry at the end of a long day to an empty refrigerator and expect to put a healthy meal on the table. You need to have healthy, prepared options at the ready so that you can quickly put together a healthy and satisfying meal. When you are in a pinch, it doesn't take long to grill or bake a chicken breast and steam a side of healthy vegetables. Resist the urge to toss in a frozen pizza when you are low on time. Sometimes it can be just as quick to toss together a big dinner salad and put some quality protein, such as last night's leftover chicken, on top.

If you will be away from home for any meal during the day, try to pack healthy options and take your food with you if possible. Remain in control of what you are eating whenever possible. If you must eat at a restaurant or elsewhere, try to select food that is as "clean" as possible and ask for sauces and dressings on the side. Remember the guideline—fill half of your plate with fruits and vegetables, heavy on the vegetables, fill a quarter of your plate with protein, and a quarter with whole grains.

Following are some additional tips, a few of which were mentioned back in *Step Seven* where we discussed time management techniques. They are worth re-mentioning as they will not only save you time, but will also help enhance your ability to serve healthy, home-cooked food even on the busiest day.

- Plan your meals for the week and shop all in one day. Knowing exactly what you are going to eat on any given day and having all of the ingredients on hand will take away the stress of having to figure it out or stop at the store at the last minute.

- Get a crock pot. Spend fifteen minutes prepping in the morning and come home to a warm, home-cooked meal.

- Consider doing some of your meal preparation on the weekend or on an evening when you have some extra time. You could peel and chop vegetables for the week and keep them in plastic bags in the refrigerator so they are ready when needed.

- Consider preparing and freezing some meals for the week in advance. That way, if you get home late or have a rushed evening, you can pull something home-cooked and healthy out of the freezer and have dinner ready in a flash.

You are much more likely to succeed in cooking and eating healthy, home-cooked meals if you take a little time to plan and prepare. Remember, you are in control.

_____Y🍵UR TURN_____

What tips will you use to make healthier meals?

What make-ahead tips will you use to prepare your meals?

Plan your menu for the coming week, including breakfast, lunch, snacks, and dinner.

Write your grocery list and shop.

Chop and prepare as much as possible in advance.

Enjoy your healthy food!

_____

_____

_____

_____

_____

_____

_____

_____

_____

_____

_____

_____

_____

_____

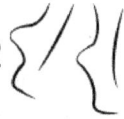

Rest

Sleep is that golden chain
that ties health and
our bodies together.

-Thomas Dekker

In our busy lives, it seems that the one thing we sacrifice most when we need additional time is our sleep. Sleep can seem like a luxury. You may feel that sleeping is taking time away from all of the other things you have to do or want to do. Completing that project or catching up on social media may seem more important than catching your zzzz's, but that couldn't be further from the truth. Sleep is productive and necessary to your health and well-being.

Lack of sleep could also affect your weight. As you sleep, your body is managing processes that control your blood sugar and which regulate feelings of hunger and satiety. Now that you are getting more exercise, sleep is more crucial than ever. If you are sleep deprived you might decide to hit the snooze and skip your workout in the morning, or be too tired to do it later in the day. Being well rested not only gives you more energy and stamina so that you can exercise, sleep also helps your body to recover from exercise. During deep sleep, your blood pressure drops and your brain activity slows. This allows additional blood to flow to your muscles, delivering oxygen and nutrients for healing and growth.

When you don't get enough sleep, you simply feel terrible. You might have body aches. You are more likely to be grumpy and short tempered. You might also become more sensitive and emotional and be less resilient in stressful situations. It can be difficult to concentrate when you are not well rested; your brain is foggy and simple tasks take longer to perform.

When you are overly tired, you might be tempted to compensate for your lack of sleep with caffeine and sugar. All of the sudden, it is more difficult to pass up that sugary coffee drink and doughnut. Your body is tired and stressed and is craving comfort, so you are more likely to grab comfort food like chips or cookies.

If you are staying up too late, chances are that you are late night snacking as well. So not only are you depriving yourself of healthful, restorative sleep, but you are also packing in extra calories. Then you go to bed on a full stomach and could be kept awake by stomach discomfort or heartburn. It is a vicious cycle.

How Much Sleep Do I Really Need?

According to the National Sleep Foundation, most adults need between seven and nine hours of sleep each night ("How Much Sleep Do We Really Need?"). You may need slightly more or less depending on your lifestyle and level of activity. Below are the recommendations based on age.

Newborn (0-3 months)	14 – 17 hours
Infant (4-11 months)	12 – 15 hours
Toddler (1-2 years)	11 – 14 hours
Pre-Schooler (3-5 years)	10 – 13 hours
School Age (6-13 years)	9 – 11 hours
Teen (14-17 years)	8 – 10 hours
Adult (18-64 years)	7 – 9 hours
Older Adult (>65 years)	7 – 8 hours

Aim for consistency, trying to get your required number of hours each night. Strive to go to bed and wake up at the same time every day. This will help to regulate your sleep cycles and could help you to sleep better.

Catching Up On Sleep

How many times have you run yourself ragged during the week and then promised to "catch up" on your sleep over the weekend? It's not a good plan. First of all, bedtime and wake time consistency is important in establishing a healthy sleep cycle. Second, a Harvard Medical study found that, "even when you sleep an extra ten hours to compensate for sleeping only six hours a night for up to two weeks, your reaction times and ability to focus is worse than if you had pulled an all-nighter," ("You Can't 'Catch Up On Sleep'").

Waking Up Happy

Our bodies were designed to wake up naturally when we are well rested with the light of the new day. Okay, stop laughing. Chances are that on most days you have to get up earlier than you might like to meet your work or family obligations. How you wake can be important. Getting jolted awake by a buzzing alarm or blasting radio can give you an instant shock of stress before your day even begins. The first order of business is to rethink your alarm. If you haven't already smashed it, toss out that annoying alarm clock. Consider waking up to light therapy instead with the help of a wake-up light. A wake-up light brightens gradually over a period of minutes and wakes you with gentle, natural sounds. You wake up peacefully and naturally.

In addition to light therapy, there are other ways you can train yourself to wake more naturally. The first is to go to bed at a consistent time which will allow you to get your necessary hours of sleep and wake rested and naturally. So if you need seven hours of sleep and must get up at 6:00a.m., you will want to be in bed and ready for sleep by 11:00p.m.

When you wake, stretch your muscles before you even get out of bed. Take a lesson from your dog or cat. Ever watch how they wake up? They stretch their legs and arch their backs and get their blood flowing before they get up.

When you get out of bed, open the curtains or go outside in

the morning light. The natural light will help to regulate your body clock and wake you fully.

Sleep Quality

Quality of sleep is just as important as the number of hours you get. If you are frequently tossing and turning or waking up in the middle of the night, you are not getting restful sleep. Sleep has four stages. Stage 1 is the act of falling asleep and entering light sleep. Stage 2 is the onset of sleep, when your body temperature drops and you become disengaged from your surroundings. Stages 3 and 4 are the deepest and most restorative phases of sleep, when your body repairs itself. If sleep is cut short or interrupted, your body doesn't have time to complete all of the phases needed for muscle repair, memory consolidation, and the release of hormones that regulate growth and appetite.

You can improve the quality of your sleep. Here are a few tips for falling asleep and staying there.

- Limit your caffeine intake. If you must have caffeine, limit it to the morning. Try a calming herbal tea in the evening.
- Keep your body hydrated, but try to avoid drinking large quantities of water in the evening that might keep you up and running to the bathroom.
- Keep your bedroom cool and dark and free from electronics. Above all, do not take your phone or any device into the bedroom that might buzz or ping and wake you up.
- Limit screen time an hour or two before bedtime. "Researchers from Brigham and Women's Hospital

_____ Y☕UR TURN _____

Journal Your Sleep

Note your bed time.

Note what time you got up for the day.

Note how many times you woke throughout the night.

Record how you feel in the morning. Do you feel rested and ready to go? What changes might you make to sleep better tomorrow?

_____

_____

_____

_____

_____

_____

_____

_____

_____

_____

_____

_____

_____

Deep restful sleep will make you look better, feel better, and will contribute greatly to your overall health. Sweet dreams.

There will be setbacks. You may slip here and there. That's okay. Just regroup and move forward. Two steps forward and one step back still keeps you moving in the right direction.

You are not done.
You are a work in progress . . . always.

You have set goals and intentions for where you would like this journey to lead, but the journey will not end when you reach your goal. When you reach your first goal, you will set another and another to keep you on the path of health and wellness. It is so easy to stray. My objective with this book is to give you tools that you can use to reach your initial goal and then keep using to stay on track, maintain, and meet future goals.

You are prepared and moving forward on your journey to health and wellness. Always keep looking toward your goal, but more importantly, enjoy the journey. Take the time to look back and see how far you have come. Be proud of your success and hold yourself accountable for your actions. You are in control. Celebrate your success.

Thank you for sharing your journey with me. I am honored to be a part of your success.

Remember that a vehicle can't run on fumes forever and you can't get water from an empty well. You can't give your best to others if you don't first take care of yourself. You are worth the effort. It's Your Turn.

is a strong body that can climb the stairs and chase the kids around. Health is feeling peaceful and happy and satisfied with yourself and with your life. Health is showing up for your loved ones and living your life to the fullest.

It doesn't matter if you are five pounds heavier than you want to be or hundreds of pounds heavier. Most of us struggle with body image and the negative self-talk that keeps us feeling uncomfortable in our clothes and uncomfortable with ourselves.

I hope you will take this journey with me and come out of it feeling like the strong, confident woman you deserve to be. It's time to take care of you. It's your turn!

Inspiration at a Glance

The secret of change is to focus all of your energy, not on fighting the old, but on building the new.

–Socrates

You must always remember...
You are Braver than you believe,
Stronger than you seem,
and Smarter than you think.

–Christopher Robin

It is never too late to be
what you might have been.

–George Elliott

Start where you are.
Use what you have.
Do what you can.

–Arthur Ashe

The only person you are destined to become
is the person you decide to be.

–Ralph Waldo Emerson

Setting goals is the first step in turning
the invisible into the visible.

–Tony Robbins

Sometimes your only available transportation
Is a Leap of Faith.

–Margaret Shepard

The most difficult thing is the decision to act.
The rest is merely tenacity.

–Amelia Earhart

Refusing to ask for help when you need it
is refusing someone the chance to be helpful.

–Rick Ocasek

Time is the most valuable coin in your life. You and you
alone will determine how that coin will be spent. Be careful
that you do not let other people spend it for you.

–Carl Sandburg

The

Contemporary
Phrase Book

Rebecca Andrews

The Contemporary Phrase Book

Table of Contents

Introduction

The concept for this book was born many years ago during an in-depth conversation with fellow writers who, like myself, were floundering in a sea of frustration. There was no source for what we were looking for: descriptive phrases that related to the contemporary market.

I'd started my own list of up-to-date tags and as time went by some friends were still searching, some were compiling their own lists, and others were ready to give up. It was then the idea for this book began to take shape.

In the years since the first printing of this book, the face of publishing has been turned upside down.

Houses and lines have merged, presses that once only offered print books have jumped on the e-book wagon. Access to a wide variety of self publishing avenues have done away with the need to take a more traditional route to see your writing published.

Whether your passion is to write a novel or an article for a newspaper or magazine, or to write a blog, it can be a challenge to come up with the right medley of words to leave your audience coming back for more.

There are only so many words in the English language. How you use and arrange those words sets you apart from other writers.

Some tags/phrases are universal no matter the venue you choose, but the right combination can do so much more than merely describe. The right choice of words can set the tone, bring the setting to life, add emotion, establish point of view, tighten the suspense or add sexual tension.

The purpose of *The Contemporary Phrase Book* is not for you to copy the phrases into your work—so don't take the easy way out. It is designed to be a useful, insightful, inspiring writer's tool. The tags found between these pages are here only to entice your imagination so you may create your own wonderfully rich descriptions. Used to prod your thought process, there is no limit to what *you* can create.

In *The Contemporary Phrase Book* I have included many categories, including some hard to find facts.

I hope you enjoy *The Contemporary Phrase Book* and use this resource to spark your creativity, inspire your imagination and kick your muse into gear. This is your tool—use it to your advantage.

Enjoy!

Rebecca

Facial Features

Face

♥~♥

Adonis	Amazonian	angelic
Aphrodite	Apollo	Aristocratic
baboon	baby-faced	big-boned
bird-like	blood-hound	bonny
boyish	bug-eyed	bullet-head
careworn	cherubic	chinless
chipmunk	chiseled	comely
craggy	crow's feet	cupid
deformed	delicate	dimpled
disfigured	distinguished	doll
dour	droopy	egg-shaped
elegant	ethereal	exotic
feline	fierce	fish
gap-toothed	gaunt	ghoulish
girlish	gnome-like	gorilla
hag	haggard	handsome
heart-shaped	hideous	high-cheekbones
hollowed	homely	insect-like
jaundiced	laugh-lines	leathery
liver-spotted	low-forehead	misshapen
Neanderthal	Nordic	Nymph
Oriental	other-worldly	oval
owlish	pig-nosed	pin-head
pixie-faced	Polynesian	rat-faced

13

regal

round

slack-jawed

sweet

repulsive

rugged

sleepy-eyed

symmetrical

roguish

sculpted

square-jawed

Ears

♥~♥~♥~♥~♥~♥~♥~♥~♥~♥~♥~♥~♥~♥~♥~♥~♥~♥

big

dangly

frostbitten

pierced

small

cauliflower (wrestler's) ear

deaf

hairy

pink or red

Vulcan or elfin

flopping

large-lobed

protruding

Eyebrows

♥~♥~♥~♥~♥~♥~♥~♥~♥~♥~♥~♥~♥~♥~♥~♥~♥~♥

angled

bent

colored

dark

high

over tweezed

patchy

scaly

shaved

tattooed

tweezed

arched

bleached

cottony

dirty

joined

over waxed

pierced

scarred

strips

thick

uni-brow

bald

bushy

curved

furry

lined

pale

plucked

shaped

symmetrical

tinted

unruly

Noses

♥~♥

aquiline	Arabian	boxer's
broad and flattened	broken, misshapen	bulbous
button	chiseled	crooked
curved, aquiline	flaring nostrils	gumdrop
Hawk	high cut nostrils	high, distinctive
hooked	hooked, curved	Jewish
long and broad	long and narrow	prissy
prominent	red and enlarged	Roman
skewed	small and (*dainty/round*)	
snub	turned up	

Teeth

♥~♥

buck teeth	corn-kernelled	crooked
dentures	gap-toothed	glistening
horse-like	jagged	pearly
saw-toothed	small	snaggle-toothed
tobacco stained	white	yellow

Facial Expressions

General

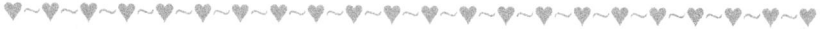

arrogant	a long, searching look
beamed with joy	face a dark mask
face hardening	flushing with indignation
frigid stare	furtive look
green eyes narrowed	his nostrils flared
incriminating look	lips curling with disgust
peered down her nose	pompous
regarded him quizzically	sidelong glance
slow, appraising glance	troubled look
withering stare	wounded look

a muscle in his clenched jaw spasmed

an ominous, thunderous expression on his face

carefully not meting her eyes, he bobbed an awkward nod

caught (*his/her*) breath at (*his/her*) grin, (*one/ two/twin*) dimple(s) deepened (*his/her*) cheek(s)

closed (*his/her*) eyes tightly and swallowed

cool calm bad ass expression

could see the fury burning hot and wild inside (*him/her*)

dark lashes half lowered over (*his/her*) eyes

expression one of supreme satisfaction

emotions played out on (*his/her*) face

expression pulled into lines of weary acceptance

eyes wide behind a thick layer of mascara

faced him with a defiant lift of her chin

face slack with surprise

found (*his/her*) expression hard to read

frustrated and annoyed, (*he/she*) shook (*his/her*) head

genuine surprise on her face

giving him a warning look he couldn't miss

guarded eyes and a slow to surface smile

had a no nonsense look about (*him/her*) that said (*he/she*) was accustomed to taking charge

her beautiful exotic face composed

her expression smoothed with obvious control

her expression was mutinous

her face expectant

his expression a furious grimace

her expression dark and rebellious

(*his/her*) elegant nose wrinkled

(*his/her*) expression revealed nothing of what (*he/she*) was thinking

his expression (*torn/twisting with indecision*)

mocked (*him/her*) with a look

peered over her rhinestone glasses

regarded (*critically/snootily/curiously/quizzically*)

scowled down at her furiously

she looked good with temper flaring in her eyes, coloring her cheeks

simply shook her head, eyes hauntingly dark with some unnamed emotion

sheer outraged amazement filled (*his/her*) expression

stony stillness of his facial expression turned his lips up in what could only be called a smirk

tanned face contorted in concentration

tension tightened the delicate features of her face

the look on (*his/her*) face changed to one of horrific disbelief as comprehension dawned

the look on (*his/her*) face was pure hatred

tossed him a sheepish look

turned (*his/her*) lips up in what could only be called a smirk

with a grin (*he/she*) nodded

worry darkened the color of (*his/her*) expression

wrinkled her pretty nose at him

Brows

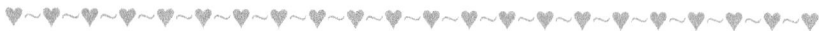

a frown darkened his brow/his frown darkened

a frown snapped between her brows

arched a brow mockingly

(*black*) brows lifted lightly at the familiarity

both eyebrows were pierced and sported gold hoops

brows and lashes like brown mink

brows (*arched in clear amusement/creased in concentration*)

brows dark and foreboding

brows lifted, he drew back to study her face

brows (*rose/raised*) in question

cocked a brow at her silence

crossed her arms and raised an amused eyebrow

dark slash of brows

eyebrows drew together in a scowl

eyebrows shot up and looked at her in (*alarm/surprise*)

eyebrows that rose and fell with more expression than some could voice

fine delicately arched brows knitted as (*he/she*) studied...

(*gray/brown*) eyebrows rose over the tops of wire-rimmed glasses

(*his/her*) brows lifted questioningly

his brow(s) lowered (*broodingly/ominously*)

his eyebrows drew together in a scowl

(*his/her*) forehead creased into a frown

irritation pinched between his dark brows

lifted an all-knowing, judgmental eyebrow

lifted (*a/one*) (*single/firmly arched*) brow easily

lifted one dark brow and grinned at (*him/her*)

long, thick lashes, darker than her pale hair

neatly plucked eyebrows slammed together

one slender brow arched in amusement

raised a doubting brow that all but called (*him/her*) a liar

smooth plane of his brow

the aggressive slash of his eyebrows

the dark wings of his eyebrows lifting fractionally

the knowing arch of his brow creased in concentration

the sweep of (*his/her*) (*dark/color*) lashes against (*his/her*) cheeks

(*thick/thin*) brows that darted like wings

winged brows dipped together over the bridge of her nose

Mouth, Chin, Jaw

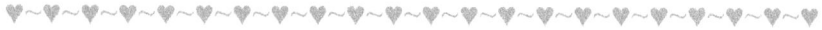

♥~♥

cleft chin	double chin	cruel
cupid's bow	disapproval	firm
flabby/fleshy	frown	full, ripe lips
heavy jaw	humorous	lantern jaw
lush bottom lip	puckered	receding chin
sassy mouth	sensuous	stubborn
square jaw	wattled	

a flat mole just below her bottom lip

a mouth created to destroy a (*man's/woman's*) (*control/sanity*)

carefully (*he/she*) closed (*his/her*) mouth

chewed on her luscious, pink bottom lip

deep dimple to the (*left/right*) of (*his/her*) mouth

downed the liquor in one swallow

full mouth set in a grim line

grinned and let out a long, low whistle

her chin quivered and she swallowed hard

her full lips thinned in anger

her lips (*wide and lush/full/rosy pink*)

his chin just the right amount of stubborn, his jaw line still sharp

(*his/her*) jaw (*flexed/tightened*) in frustration

his jaw hadn't seen a razor today

(*his/her*) lips hovered just over (*his/hers*)

his strong mouth was pressed into a smirk

lips cruelly sensual

lips folded thoughtfully

lips took on a mutinous tilt

lips that begged to be kissed without saying a word

lips that half pouted and half mocked

lips wide and full

lush mouth that protested a little too much

made a small 'o' with those pouty lips

mouth created to destroy a (*man's/woman's*) control

(*mouth/jaw*) tightened

ran his tongue over his long, left canine tooth

she (*licked/moistened*) her lips

smile held a hint of smugness

strong line of his jaw tightened

talented mouth and even more talented fingers

teeth, perfectly even and white against his bronzed good looks

the fierce angle of her chin

the fullness of her mouth

top lip full, bottom thin

well-defined kissable mouth

wide full lips that drove a man wild

Smiles

angelic	blissful	brave
broad	Cheshire cat	closed mouth
condescending	conspiratorial	coy
crafty	cruel	curt
defiant	demure	devastating
dirty	dreamy	embarrassed
forced	genuine	gleeful

gracious	grimace	guarded
humiliated	hurtful	incredulous
incriminating	involuntary	inward
knowing	lifeless	leer
lacking emotion	lopsided	malicious delight
mocking	nasty	nervous
obligatory	patronizing	phony
pinched	polite	pretentious
salacious	self-conscious	sheepish
spiteful	spastic	tight
thin	triumphant	twitchy
victorious	wicked	whistle of discovery

a crooked smile that hinted at a hidden wild side

a disarming grin

a do-me smile

a feminine little sneer curled her lips

a grin quirked (*his/her*) sensual lips

a lazy taunting smile slid from one side of his beard-stubbled jaw to the other

a masculine mouth twitched at one end into a wry grin

an unwilling smile tugged at (*his/her*) lips

a pirate grin that glittered in his dark eyes

a pleased sound escaped (*him/her*)

a (*shameless/sheepish*) (*grin/smile*)

a sinister half-smile curved (*his/her*) lips

a smile crinkled the corners of (*his/her*) eyes

a smile of pure sin

a smile quirked (*his/her*) too sensual mouth

a slow smile slowly tipped up one corner of his mouth

a smug, mocking smile

a sudden luminous smile lit her face

a surprising wry edge to his mouth

a warm, friendly, country-boy grin

a wicked, feral smile curved his lips

a wry grin split the somberness of his face

asked with the smallest curve of his lips

bared teeth in a cold little smile

beaming at (*him/her*)

(*broad/good humored*) grin split his face

Cheshire cat smile stretched wide

contained a spark of eroticism

corner of his sensual mouth lifted in a lazy, half smile

deftly covered (*his/her*) laughter with a cough

devil-be-damned/shit-eating grin

disbelieving frown

expression pure cunning as (*he/she*) stepped toward (*him/her*)

face broke into a grin, light and fierce, his combat grin

felt a smile of pure masculine pleasure spread across his face

flashed a (*sweet smile/superior grin*)

flashed that famous grin, the one that had (*men/women/
groupies*) following (*him/her*)

framed by inviting dimples that enchanted (*him/her*)

gave (*him/her*) a (*nervous/mocking*) smile

grin widened to show (*his/her*) white teeth

grinned his good-ole-boy grin

grinned (*smugly/like a wolf*)

grinned sheepishly and cleared his throat

grinned smugly

grinned to put (*him/her*) at ease

grinned with a distinctly male satisfaction

had a repertoire of smiles for every occasion

(*he/she*) flashed (*him/her*) a sexy, wicked smile

(*he/she*) (*smiled like a saint/smothered*) a (*grin/smile*)

her lips slipped into a charming flirtatious grin

her lips tightened in irritation

he smiled his seductive smile and her hormones did an excited little dance

he smiled, offered his hand and his name

her smile changed her face, softened it, added a touch of vulnerability

his answering grin flashed white against the shadows

his face broke into a grin, light and fierce

his features softened with a boyish charm

his grin both boyish and roguish

his grin full of hungry anticipation

his grin revealed blood stained canines

(*his/her*) grin was not the least bit apologetic

(*his/her*) face beamed with joy

(*his/her*) lips twitched into a shy and delighted smile

(*his/her*) mouth (*curved/grinned in amusement*)

(*his/her*) mouth curved indulgently

(*his/her*) mouth eased into a grin (*he/she*) couldn't control

(*his/her*) mouth relaxed into a sensual smile

(*his/her*) sensual mouth lifted in a lazy, half smile

(*his/her*) smile held a hint of smugness

(*his/her*) smile hinted at sex and mystery

(*his/her*) smile was filled with humor

(*his/her*) smile was (*mocking/bitter/forced*)

(*his/her*) smile was slow, naughty and completely breathtaking

his lips were sensual, firm, and curved in the hint of a smile

his smile turned his mouth into the most beautiful set of lips she'd ever seen

his smile was (*absolutely immoral/devastating*)

his smile was blatant male confidence

hugged (*him/her*) and they air kissed

irresistible and devastating

irritating, knowing smile

laughed warmly and richly

laugh lines bracketed his unsmiling mouth

lips curved in a dangerous smile

lips quirked wryly

lips stretched back over strong, white teeth

lips twisted in a tight-lipped grin

lips twitched in amusement

lips twitched at her flirtatiousness

lips twitched into a shy and delighted smile

look of (*delight/bliss/rapture*)

looked into (*his/her*) face and winked

love to wipe that smug expression off his face

mouth elegant, gracefully shaped and ready to quirk up into a smile

mouth tipped in a lazy, sexy smile

offered his best, I'm-a-nice-guy smile

pressed freshly painted lips into a seductive smile

raised one corner of his mouth

scowled melodramatically

sensually full, mobile mouth curved into a grin of sheer male confidence and superiority

sexy, arrogant mouth curved in a smile

she gave him a soft warm smile

shot him a good-natured smile and clapped an arm around his shoulders

slow (*sexy smile/half smile*)

smile played slowly around (*his/her*) lips

smiled a small, trembling smile

smiled a smile of pure sin

smiled at her and it was all she could do not to melt at his feet

smiled (*broadly/jauntily/engagingly*)

smiled, but the curve of (*his/her*) mouth had nothing to do with humor

smiled, (false gentleness/fake sweetness)

smiled (*in/with*) gloating satisfaction

smiled innocently batting her eyelashes

smiled suggestively, then ran her tongue slowly over full lips

smiled with chilling politeness

smiling, he was stunningly gorgeous

smile was devastating and without a hint of fang

smile was engaging

smile was pure sex appeal

snorted in an unladylike fashion

the seductive smile he flashed at her

thin, grim face lit with a murderous smile

two perfect dimples formed in her cheeks

whistle of discovery

whooped, slapping her knee with a hand

wide-cheeked ebony face split with a white smile

women who could resist his slow, hot smile fell for his boyish grin

wry grin split the somberness of his face

Negative Expressions

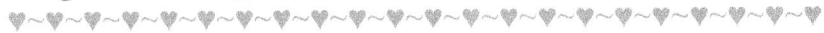

♥~♥~♥~♥~♥~♥~♥~♥~♥~♥~♥~♥~♥~♥~♥~♥~♥~♥~♥

| cleft chin | double chin | heavy jaw |
| lantern jaw | lack jawed | wattled |

a (*nasty smile/fuck you sneer*)

an angry snarl curled (*his/her*) lip

a slow, evil smile spread over his handsome face

a small frown slipping across her face

a sniff of disapproval

brutally sculpted lips curled in a cruel smile

considered his toothless smile a badge of honor

expression was pure cunning

forced a charming smile to his lips

full lips curved into a nasty smile

gave a grin in which half his teeth were missing

gave a noncommittal grunt

greeted (*him/her*) with a polite mouth-only smile

grinned with the satisfaction of the truly self-deluded

grin was (*decidedly nasty/cold and harsh*)

grinned with a tight malevolence

hang dog expression

he looked slightly wounded

(*he/she*) forced a charming smile to (*his/her*) lips

(*he/she*) frowned thoughtfully

her full lips thinned in anger

her pursed lips bespoke her lack of sympathy

her small teeth tugged briefly at her full lower lip

(*he/she*) sneered at (*him/her*)

his (*brown/gray*) eyes were as ruthless and remote as they'd been the day she'd betrayed him

(*his/her*) expression fierce, furious

(*his/her*) expression twisting with indecision

(*his/her*) expression was mutinous

(*his/her*) expression was troubled

(*his/her*) intense scowl

(*his/her*) smile faded

(*his/her*) lip curled in disgust

his lips twisted painfully

kept his face hard and unyielding

lines of his face etched with deep concern

lips curving downward, to frame his black goatee

lips pressed together in stubborn anger

lips tightened in irritation

looked slightly wounded

look of ice cold fury on (*his/her*) face

mouth flattened into a (*hard/uncompromising*) line

pasted a polite smile on her face

pout/pouting

pressed (*his/her*) lips tightly together

slack jawed

small frown slipping across her face

smile faded from his eyes, and his mouth

smiled, but it never reached his cold, (*black/dark*) eyes

smile was cold, ruthless, (*mocking, bitter*)

smiled with (*malice/maliciously*)

snarl of agony

sneered at her hatefully

the corners of his (*beautiful/mobile/sensuous*) mouth tugged downward as he stared at her

the easy smile dropped from his face

the expression on (*his/her*) face was shadowed with suspicion

the look on (*his/her*) face anything but welcoming

thin, nearly cruel lips drew flat over his teeth

tried to smile but it fell flat

usually smiling gaze went dead sober

Feminine Traits

Body

♥~♥

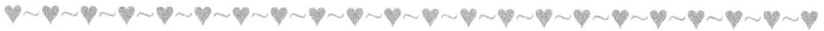

attractive	beautiful	charming
comely	curvy	dainty
delicate	elegant	exquisite
fair	fragile of bone	graceful
lively	lovely	lush curves
neat	nimble	pretty
ravishing	reed-like	regal
ripe curves	shapely	slender
small boned	soft	statuesque
symmetrical	tall	trim
vivacious	wild beauty	

a delicacy about her body
all sleek curves and finely toned muscle
amazingly stacked
a petite (*blonde/brunette*) with very large breasts
a tiny sprite of a woman
average wasn't a word that could ever be used to describe her
beautiful, slim and leggy
beautiful woman with a (*bright mind/quick temper/soft heart*)
(*blonde/brunette*), big-breasted, shallow

could plainly see her body was (*curved/lush*) in all the right places

curvy, womanly with a small waist, rounded hips and a neat little triangle of pubic hair

elegant young woman

ethereal, other worldly air about her

had a body that pushed all his buttons in a very big way

her stance was uncompromising

her T-shirt clung to her full figure enticingly

incredibly feminine with a delicate bone structure

leggy (*blonde/brunette*), with hungry eyes

legs were long, her jeans slightly loose on her hips and thighs

lithe and young, with a beauty only surpassed by her intelligence

loose limbed and graceful

luscious curves fitting snugly in a short denim skirt

incredibly feminine with delicate bone structure

one of those rare women who was beautiful without being obvious

petite, curvy (*dark mahogany/coffee toned*) skin

pride and absolute confidence in her stance

she looked like walking sex

she was too young, too pretty, too desperately hopeful

small, slender etched with muscle and grace

smooth slender thighs

soft-as-sin curves

such an itty-bitty thing at barely five foot

supple lithe limbs

tall, slender with deep (*color*) eyes and ebony hair that fell in thick waves past her hips

tall, willowy form

tan, slim dressed in the height of fashion

the (*color*) suit she wore showcased her endless legs and hugged her generous breasts

the lovely girl was now a beautiful woman

the top of her head lined up with his chin

tight denim jeans molded to her hips and thighs

wore faded, curve-hugging jeans

Negative

awkward	clumsy	effeminate
frail	graceless	homely
repugnant	repulsive	spare
thin	ungainly	ugly
unwomanly		

Face

adorable	angelic	attractive
charming	cunning	cute
dainty	delicate	delicate nose
delicate of feature	exquisite	gorgeous
graceful	handsome	lovely
lush bottom lip	long slender neck	pink lips
pleasing	pout	pretty
ravishing	rosebud mouth	sensuous lips
strong square jaw	stubborn little chin	stunning

a sensuous, delicate sculpture of high cheekbones

baby smooth skin, perfect, delicately shaped features

biting her lip nervously

cheekbones high, mouth wide and well shaped

delicate porcelain doll features

face porcelain smooth against her (*brunette/dark*) hair

face was a contorted mixture of misery and embarrassment

face was bewitching, beguiling

fine straight nose, just a tiny tilt at the (*end/tip*)

forced his attention away from her sexy mouth

full lips plastered with kiss-me-or-die (*red/pink/mocha*) lipstick

full square face, with high, proud cheekbones

glasses tilted on her straight, little nose

had a face that didn't need softening—it was already soft enough

had a warm tawny complexion

heart-stoppingly gorgeous

her beauty held a sweetness to which he was powerfully drawn

her cheeks flushed

her (*face/expression*) was pure determination

her small straight nose, fit her heart shaped face

lashes laying on her cheeks were very long and as dark as her hair

long slender neck

mouth always tilted into a smile, eyes always merry

perfectly straight, perfectly white teeth

perfect olive skin

prominent cheekbones

sculpted cheekbones, a (*sinful mouth/sensuous lips*)

she had skin like magnolia's

she was a pretty little thing, as finely made as an expensive porcelain figurine

smooth parchment of her skin

smooth, porcelain skin

straight nose and a wide full mouth

unruly splash of freckles

wide, full lipped mouth

young, simple face, all curves and rosy skin

Hair

💗~💗~💗~💗~💗~💗~💗~💗~💗~💗~💗~💗~💗~💗~💗~💗~💗~💗~💗~💗

a cap of glossy (*brown*) hair

a tangle of (*red/auburn*) hair spilled over her shoulders

a wall of damp, (*cinnamon/blonde*) colored hair

(*auburn and ginger/grayish*) hue of her hair

(*black/brown*) hair fanned out like a cloud of dark silk

(*blonde/brunette*) hair cut into a feathery looking (*style/wisps*) that (*framed/surrounded*) her pale face

(*blonde/red*) hair piled high in an (*ugly/outdated*) style

(*blonde/black/auburn*) hair tumbled around her flushed face

braided hair pulled into a ball at the nape of her neck

cascaded in riotous waves from a (*silver/gold*) clip

coal black, cut in short, sassy spikes

curled wildly against her shoulders

(*dark brown*) hair escaping her ponytail in glossy strands around her face

(*dark/fiery*) hair swirled around her shoulders

framing her face like a pool of glossy silk

frigid breeze combed reckless fingers through her hair

hair a gleaming mane of six different shades of (*gold/red*)

hair (*fell/tumbled*) loosely (*around/to*) her shoulders, ended in the middle of her back

hair formed a perfect halo around about her head

hair on her sex was darker than the hair on her head

hair rolled up in pink plastic curlers

hair swept up and pinned primly in a French roll

hair (*swept up/pulled*) into a (*stern knot/bun*) at the (*back/ top*) of her (*head/skull*)

hair that reached past her waist

hair the color of corn-silk

hair the taffy color of moonshine whiskey

hair tumbled around her flushed face

hair was long, (*blonde*) and straight

head full of disobedient curls

her dark hair was cut boyishly short

long brown hair that lay like thick ribbons around her slender body

long hair plaited down her back

long hair hung in (*loose, thick*) waves

long, shiny (*jet black/blonde/brown*) hair (*curled/danced*) in loose wisps on her (*shoulders/along*) her neck and throat

long strands of (*blonde/red/jet black*) hair had escaped from the bun at the back of her head

loved the way it tickled his face when she was over him

newly washed, set and sprayed, it wouldn't have moved in a (*storm/tornado*)

no perm or fake highlights to ruin what she'd been born with (*pale flaxen/blonde*) hair fell around her shoulders and down her back like a mantle of silk

pale hair cut short and sleek

ran a hand through her short, (*reddish-gold/sandy brown*) hair

(*red/brown/black*) hair hung in little ringlets down to her shoulders

(*red/brown/black*) hair spilled over his chest like an ocean of fragrant silk

ruler straight bangs

(*rusty-red/brown/black*) hair elegantly styled beneath a pillbox hat with a short veil

(*color*) hair fanned out on the pillow

same big hair as her high school days

saw her fingers rake through that glorious, thick, (*color*) hair

several strands dangled haphazardly around her face

shimmering (*copper/red*) hair streaked with gold

short (*blonde/red*) curls bobbed

shoulder length, frizzy brown hair

silky shoulder length hair, an eye-catching (*silver-gray/jet black*)

(*snow white/gray*) hair styled close to her head/sleekly styled

tendrils of jaw length (*coffee-brown*) hair

touched a bejeweled hand to her immaculately coifed hair

waist length (*black/brown/blonde*) hair partially hiding her face like a thick, ebony curtain

wealth of thick, silky hair framed a delicate, oval face

wealth of tight (*strawberry-blonde/light brown*) curls that cascaded without order

wore her hair with no bangs to soften her face

wore her (*honey-brown/light blonde*) hair swept up

Additional Descriptions
♥~♥~♥~♥~♥~♥~♥~♥~♥~♥~♥~♥~♥~♥~♥~♥~♥~♥~♥

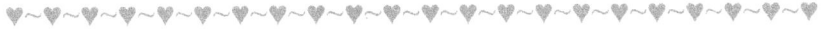

admirable	alluring	angelic
appealing	attractive	beguiling
bewitching	bonny	brilliant
charming	captivating	comely
cute	dazzling	delightful
divine	elegant	enchanting
enticing	engaging	enthralling
eye-catching	exquisite	fair
fascinating	fetching	fine
glamorous	gorgeous	graceful
grand	handsome	inviting
lovely	magnificent	marvelous
mesmerizing	pleasing	pretty
radiant	ravishing	refined
resplendent	splendid	striking
stunning	tantalizing	tempting

a bone-thin, sucked dry older woman
a five (*or six*)-foot woman with a wild mane of curly, (*jet-black/ dark brown*) hair
a gait guaranteed to snag a man's attention and hold it
a haughty (*thirty/forty*)-something (*blonde/brunette*) in an
alabaster skin flawless as virgin snow
all curves and attitude in a small package
appearance spoke of wealth and breeding
armed to the teeth make up
a serene, quiet sort of beauty
black leather skirt that barely covered her essentials
bronzed skin unblemished and smooth, vibrant and healthy

coke bottle glasses sitting askew on her nose

cool elegance and private school accent

crisp business suit and high heels

cultivated an image among the party crowd of being (*loose/ easy/unattainable*)

dainty silver rings circled her painted toes

demure, very proper (*town librarian/school marm*)

each finger adorned with a ring

(*earrings/diamond studs*) (*sparkled/winked*) at her earlobes in the florescent light

even tempered and logical

expensive designer suit and high heels

first-class brain and a snotty (*attitude/personality*)

fleshy cheeks framed an oversized nose

full lips painted a shiny (*red/pink*)

fury etched on her intelligent face

hard headed, smart and sassy

heavy-set woman with teased (*red/black*) hair

her appearance spoke of wealth and breeding

her curves didn't need the help of fancy clothes, they made themselves known no matter what she wore

her entire body felt more sensitive from her pregnancy

her tongue stroked her lips with a soft, sensual lick

her upturned face was pale

incredible gold-velvet skin

moonlight shimmered over her white skin, lending it a faint exotic cast

played a leading role in every straight man's x-rated fantasies

she oozed southern-belle charm

she was a (*feisty beauty/spitfire/steamy–eyed/saucy mix of contradictions*)

silky, flaxen skin glowed against her wedding gown

sleepiness just one more of the many changes pregnancy was making in her body

soaked to the bone she looked like a waterlogged urchin

strong unbending will

sunglasses pushed over her head

surgical nips and tucks kept her hovering at (*age*)

tanned a deep russet brown

too straight-laced for anything devious or treacherous

unexpected grace that softened her face

Create Your Own Tags!!!

Masculine Traits

Body

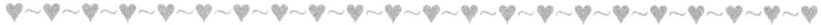

able-bodied	athletic	beefy
big	brawny	broad-shouldered
bulky	dense	enormous
great	hard	hardy
hearty	heavily built	hefty
huge	husky	immense
large	massive	muscular
mighty	oversized	powerful
powerfully built	prodigious	robust
solid	stalwart	stocky
stout	strapping	strong
strongly-built	sturdy	thick
thickset	tough	well-built

bare to the waist	clean cut, athletic
great wide shoulders	his regal aura
lean muscular physique	long heavily muscled legs
massive biceps flexing	numerous scars
six-foot-three and solid muscle	strongly masculine
tall, bronze frame	tall, lanky build

a bit of male animal just under the surface

a body designed purely for female pleasure

a body made perfect with the promise of hard, lean muscle

a careless charm that seemed to draw women to him

a deep gorge of spine gave rise to the thick walls of muscle on either side of it

a good cop, honest, hardworking, and straightforward

a large ebony-skinned man

a lean powerful runners body

an earthy wildness about him

a neat diamond of hair stretched over his chest

a primal masculinity

a rippling six-pack of abs any man would envy

a solid (*six-foot-three*) of Nordic blond good looks

a subtle aura that drew the glance of every female

a tall, lean figure swaggered through the open doorway

a thick, silky trail of dark hair began just above the navel and slid down into...

a trickle of sweat ran down the center of his back

a warrior who had battled hard and seen much

an amazing specimen of masculinity

an earthy wildness about him

an enormous (*African-American/Asian*) with a shaved head

an indescribable masculine aura about him

at (*six-foot-three*), very little of his body was fat

black leather chaps framed and drew attention to his crotch, covered in snug, faded denim

blatantly sexy with his bedroom eyes and roguish smile

body as impressive as the face

breadth of his heavy shoulders

broad chest beneath his crossed arms

chest tapered nicely down to a tight waist and slim hips

chiseled, he was an exquisite hunk of carved mahogany

clean shaven skin the color of shelled walnuts

close friend and card playing buddy

copper-colored skin that turned females' heads

disposition of a rattlesnake with a sore tooth

exuded a level of charismatic power

faded snug jeans that fit him all too well

golden hair dusted his forearms yet was dark beneath his arms

good-old-country boy exterior

greedy, bullying, unscrupulous SOB

hard body that beckoned with sexual promise

hard muscled thighs bulged against the material of his (*jeans, slacks*) with every ground eating stride

he looked dashing, handsome and deadly

he seemed a little rumpled, sleepy as if he'd just climbed out of bed

he stirred, a slight ripple of muscle warning of his enormous strength

he transformed from sexy man to savage beast

he was rock hard and deep to the muscle brown

hidden beneath dark chest hair, she saw small brown nipples

his arms were muscled, his stomach tapered, without an ounce of fat

his ass was tight, perfectly formed and packed with sweet muscle

his bare form radiated a threatening and well-exercised strength

his body a map of faded scars

his body exemplified everything she had come to expect of him—power, endurance and strength

his cheeks sharp and angled

his chest, a perfect set of abs covered by glistening skin

his demeanor that of a stud who'd earned the right to the title

his forehead was high and proud

his muscles bulged in perfect proportion to his height and weight

his presence even more compelling up close

his skin tanned gold and smooth

jagged scar on his (*thigh/bicep/cheek*)

jeans revealed a wiry leanness that came from years in the saddle

jeans that rode low on his lean hips, unbuttoned to reveal a hard flat belly

late forties with graying hair

leather pants showcased not only the strength of his legs, but the size of his erection

legs and butt were dusted with silky dark hair

long and lean, with broad shoulders and a wide chest

long legs, long arms, big hands

long neck, long limbs, (*sandy/light-brown*) hair

looked dashing, handsome and deadly

looked huge, powerful, very dangerous

looked like an angel of death come to call

looking like a range-tough cowboy determined to have his way

lower down on his abdomen his navel was circled with the same dark hair

lower half of his body covered in supple black leather

middle-aged man with (*sandy-brown*) hair and a trim mustache

muscles flexed and relaxed with the flow of his movements

narrow waist and lean hips

noting the breadth of his shoulders and the length of his legs

one hundred and ninety pounds (*or whatever weight*) of male frustration staring at her

plain (*white*) shirt that bulged over impressive biceps

possessed a hot sexuality that kept women coming back

possessed a magnetism that couldn't be explained with words

powerful muscles shaped his long legs and massive thighs

radiated strength, determination and heat

rippling muscles of his chest and stomach seemed the size of a mountain

short, stocky build, all muscle

shoulders bulging beneath his black T-shirt

six-two (*or whatever height*) with a reedy, wiry build

skin the color of (*midnight/walnut/coffee*)

sleek, powerful build of a finely toned athlete

slow, seductive walk

snug jeans and a shirt rolled up to the elbows

squat with thick limbs and a protruding belly

stance drew eyes to the width of his shoulders

straightening his wide shoulders

suggested strength and authority

superficial and immature, his single most recurring thought about sex

tall, overly thin (*African-American/Asian/Mexican, etc.*) man

tan cargo pants hugged his butt in an amazing fit

tanned skin and hard male muscle in motion

tattoo peeking from beneath one sleeve

tense shoulders, so strong, so durable

the air of supremacy rolled off him in waves

the force of his presence struck her anew

the long, lean lines of his body were stiff

the man had that elusive quality that drew others, even against their will

the man oozed power, authority, and raw animal sexuality

the man was as talented as he was gorgeous

the aura of confidence and competence surrounded him

torso cut into six bricks that tapered into a slim waist

trim and smooth limbed from martial arts practice

wearing jeans and a T-shirt the color of (*chocolate/coffee*) that fit his athletic body like a second skin

well-defined hips had a confident slant

well over six feet of rangy, powerful male

Negative

♥~♥

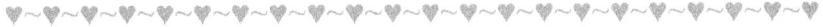

awkward	clumsy	coarse
decrepit	effeminate	emaciated
feeble	frail	gawky
ghastly	grotesque	hideous
horrible	lanky	loathsome
repellant	repugnant	repulsive
revolting	sickly	skinny
spare	thin	ungainly
unkempt	unmanly	weak

Face

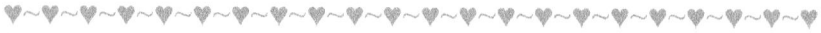

big-nosed face

blunt square face

carved

chiseled good looks

clean-cut

cut

etched with savagery

fine large nose

handsome as the devil

hard jaw

long hawkish nose

profile

rough and dangerous

sculptured

sharp-cut

sketch

stamp

well-balanced

blatant maleness

brutal lines

cast

chiseled visage

coarsely lined face

distinct

face of a saint

freshly shaven (*face/jaw*)

hard angles of his face

high forehead

perfect symmetry

quietly regal

rugged good looks

shadowed

silhouette

square jawed

stern bony mask

a bony, slightly, melancholy face

a face like a movie star and a smile that makes you want to follow him just about anywhere

a few days growth on his lean jaw

a long, narrow face broken by sharp cheekbones

a look of such profound (*sadness/thoughtfulness*)

a wild handsome face half hidden behind mirrored glasses

a work of impossible masculine beauty

angular jaw emanated power and determination

beautiful, sexy face half lit by moonlight

belly-of-a-snake white skin

chiseled (*caramel/coffee*) good looks

dark shadow stubbled his sculpted jaw

dusky skin and the contours of his face proudly proclaimed his (*Spanish/Native American/etc.*) heritage

expression on his face was stern, though fatherly

exquisite perfection brushed with a touch of wildness

face designed to make a woman whisper with lust

face had filled out, giving him a ruggedly masculine appeal

face savagely (*painted/streaked*) with (*colors*)

face too handsome for his own good

face was ruddy and ravaged by old acne scars

features spoke of maturity and self assurance

hard masculine lips formed in perfect sensuality

hawk nose, sharp cheekbones seemingly etched into stone by wind and weather

head as round as a pumpkin

he was rugged, unruly and untamed looking

high, proud cheekbones were chiseled out of a face of dark beauty

his mouth, mobile and sensual

his skin was tawny-velvet, darkly stubbled

large, stout man with round whiskered jowls

lines of worry had collected near the corners of his mouth

lively (*blue-gray*) eyes framed by wire-rimmed glasses

long and lean, moonlight accented fascinating shadows under his cheekbones

long, narrow face broken by sharp cheekbones

markedly prominent forehead

nose was too short

pleasant unassuming looks

recklessly handsome features

rugged angles, sharp (*lines/planes/high cheekbones*)

rugged-jawed poster boy for law enforcement officers

sharp featured face of planes and angles

slicked back hair and sharp, pinched features

smug, masculine arrogance

square cut jaw, wide firm mouth

that he'd lived hard and long was etched deep in his face

the last (*two/however many*) years had carved a hardness to his features

thin, narrow face, sensuous mouth and square jaw

web of lines at the corners of his eyes

Hair

♥~♥~♥~♥~♥~♥~♥~♥~♥~♥~♥~♥~♥~♥~♥~♥~♥~♥~♥

beard   five-o-clock shadow/stubble   goatee

man bun   moustache   sideburns

shaved head   soul patch

a few (*gray/white*) hairs had dared invade his temples

a mane of (*black/brown*) hair curled from his forehead to just below his ears

a prominent widow's peak

a sleek fall of (*black/brown*) hair

a small goatee and short (*black/brown*) hair

a (*thick crop of iron gray/thinning gray hair*)

a thin line of velvety dark hair arrowed downward

bald head shining like a beacon

black hair pulled back from an aristocratic face

(*black/brown*) hair streaked with gray

breeze lifting his steel-colored hair

brown streaks tangled in his silky dreads complemented his dark complexion

color of straw and stuck up at odd angles

combed shaking fingers through the few strands of hair gracing his head

crowned with a thick layer of short-cropped hair

dark and thick as devil's velvet

(*dark/blond*) hair, windswept and streaked with lighter tones

(*dark/blond*) hair (*curled/fell*) forward carelessly over his (*collar/shoulders*)

(*dark/blond*) hair laid in the sort of thick waves a woman's fingers itched to plunge into

(*dark/blond*) hair, overly long and sinfully thick, framed the hard planes of his face

diamond shape of (*black/brown*) hair that stretched from nipple to nipple on his chest

glints of (*red/blond*) in his dark, tousled hair

(*golden/dark*) hair slightly longer than fashion dictated

(*gray/brown*) hair, thick mustache and long sideburns sprinkled with salt and pepper

hair as thinly white as the moon

hair cut short with a slight bronzing at the tips

his thick, (*color)* hair was matted with sweat

jet-black and curled over his ears and the collar of his shirt

light (*brown/chestnut*) streaked by the sun

long, (*black/brown*) hair pulled back into a sleek ponytail

(neatly trimmed/short/close cropped) (brown/blond)
(hair/hair cut)

one shock of thick, *(dark/brown/black)* hair tumbled over his furrowed forehead

military short high and tight

shock of dark *(red/blond)* hair and a dimple in his left cheek

shoulder-length, *(jet black/brown/blond)* hair

slick, *(blond/etc.)* hair ever so slightly disarranged

smoothed his neat, salt-and-pepper mustache

spiky, *(light/brown/etc.)* hair had hints of chestnut and gold woven throughout

streaks of blond hair that looked as if they'd been bleached by the sun

sun-kissed tawny locks that curled

sun-streaked dark *(blond/brown/etc.)* hair

thick, *(black/brown/etc.)* hair was matted with sweat

two thin braids hung from his *(left/right/on either side of his)* temple

wet, *(black/brown)* hair was slicked back

wheat-colored hair seemed to glow in the night

Additional Descriptions

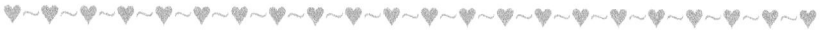

♥~♥~♥~♥~♥~♥~♥~♥~♥~♥~♥~♥~♥~♥~♥~♥~♥~♥~♥

a chaw of tobacco stuck in his cheek

a diamond stud in his left ear

a huge bear of a man

a man of mystery

a man who suffered no hesitation or inhibitions

a man who was one-hundred percent okay with lust

a naughty rambunctious streak

arrogance and entitlement of aristocracy

a way about him that commanded respect

an amazing specimen of masculinity

bare feet sticking out under the table

boots scuffed and crusted with dirt

brooding sexuality swirled around him

careless charm that seemed to draw women to him

cold, icy fortress of a man who guarded himself carefully

dressed in a dark button-down shirt and slacks

dressed in an expensive western-cut suit and cowboy boots

dressed in fatigues and army boots

dressed in shorts and a chest hugging T-shirt

extraordinarily macho reputation

faded denim bagging over his thin torso

faded wrangler jeans with battered, low heeled boots

had a noticeable belly

had a proud lineage

he was a balding little man

he wasn't a bad looking guy, in a linebacker sort of way

laid back, sweet talking, sexy as hell

looked dark and dangerous

looked tired, edgy and beaten down

overachiever, preferred the label playboy

part of the seen and be seen crowd

plain T-shirt, plastered to his torso by sweat

prided himself on individuality

prime example of raw male power

pudgy, balding, rumpled man in a wrinkled raincoat

raw mysterious power emanated from him

scrumptious piece of eye candy

sexy as homemade sin

sleeves rolled back, revealing strong forearms

smooth-talking shallow playboy

stunning male power and strength

struggled to be his own boss in all ways

surged up in one graceful ripple of animalistic strength

the gait of a man comfortable in his own skin

the solid black he'd chosen only accentuated his aura of sexuality

there was no insignia, no rank, no markings on his camouflage gear

wickedly alluring

wide, gold wedding band on his ring finger

wire-rimmed reading glasses in the pocket of his sport (*coat/jacket*)

worked his fingers into the muscles at the back of his neck

Body Types

Female

♥~♥~♥~♥~♥~♥~♥~♥~♥~♥~♥~♥~♥~♥~♥~♥~♥~♥~♥~♥

athletic	buxom	compact
curvaceous	delicate	diminutive
fit	full-figured	hourglass curves
lavishly endowed	leggy	lithe
petite	sleek	slim
slinky	stacked	statuesque
svelte	tall	thin
willowy		

Male

♥~♥~♥~♥~♥~♥~♥~♥~♥~♥~♥~♥~♥~♥~♥~♥~♥~♥~♥~♥

burly	chiseled/defined pecs	
iron-muscled	lanky	lean
long-legged	rippling	rock-hard
rugged	sinewy	strapping
toned	towering	wiry

Additional Descriptions

♥~♥~♥~♥~♥~♥~♥~♥~♥~♥~♥~♥~♥~♥~♥~♥~♥~♥~♥~♥

Amazonian	barrel-chested	beefy
beer-belly	big-as-a-bull/ox	blubbery
brawny	chubby	colossal
fat/doughy	gaunt	haggard
hairy	hunched	love-handles
lumpy	middle-aged	midget
obese/fleshy	paunchy	pear-shaped
plump	portly	pot-bellied
pudgy	roly-poly	runt
scrawny		

Body Parts

Arms and Hands

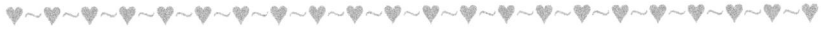

♥~♥

arthritic elbow	banged up hands	bony hands/fingers
calloused fingers	chapped hands	clammy hands
claw-like fingers	corded arms	fingernail
fist	flabby arms	forearm
gnarled fingers	greasy-oily hands	hairy hands
hand (*left and right*)	hands like hams	long, delicate hands
manicured hands	palm	pudgy hands
red, chapped hands	stick like arms	stubby fingers
thumb	work-worn hands	wrestler's arms

finger- (*index finger/middle/little/ring/pinky*)

Head, Shoulders, and Chest

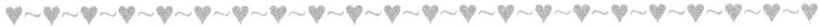

♥~♥

barrel-chested	cheek	chin
chiseled pecs	defined pecs	ear
eye	eyebrow	eyelash
forehead	hair/hairless/ hairy	head
jaw	lip	mouth
neck	nose	nostril
shoulder	throat	tongue
tooth/teeth		

Legs and Feet

♥~♥~♥~♥~♥~♥~♥~♥~♥~♥~♥~♥~♥~♥~♥~♥~♥~♥

ankle	calf	foot/feet
heel	hips	knee
leg	shin	thigh
toe/big toe/little toe	toenail	

Trunk or Torso

♥~♥~♥~♥~♥~♥~♥~♥~♥~♥~♥~♥~♥~♥~♥~♥~♥~♥

abs	back	beer-bellied
blubbery	bottom	chest
chiseled stomach	cut abdomen	flabby
fleshy	iron stomach	love-handles
paunchy	plump	pot-bellied
rippling	spare-tire	toned
middle aged spread	washboard	

Body Movements

General

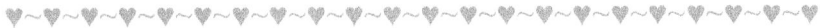

apologetic shrug

arranged his face in a scowl as he turned

bowed from the waist in a courtly old-fashioned gesture

bracing her hands on either side of her, caging her in with his powerful body

carefully shielded her with his body

confident deadly swagger of a man who knew he had no equal

crossed (*his/her*) (*jean clad/mile-long*) legs

dabbed at the perspiration beading (*his/her*) brow

did a fast dip and spin, then rocked her hips to the beat

dragging the (*curvaceous beauty/sex kitten*) with him

gave a loose-muscled shrug

he shrugged, a graceful movement of one muscular shoulder

he shrugged his powerful shoulders

jerking off his bloodied surgical uniform, he left the OR

leaned against the wall and breathed deep

long legs felt leaden as she moved

long legs stretched out on the desk top in front of him

moved with a freedom and unconsciousness

moved with such economy—an almost fluid grace

movements restrained and controlled

one sandal dangled playfully off her big toe

powerful arms crossed over his chest

powerful body filling the doorway

pressing one hand over her heart, as if that would still it's
frantic pounding

pushed away from the (*car/truck/fence*) and came toward her

rigid lift of his shoulders

sat there like some complicated mix of mischievous girl and
sexy, earth woman

sauntered toward her, hands thrust in the pockets of his worn
jeans

settled his long, thin torso into the vinyl seat

she stiffened, whirled to face him

shoulders slumped

shoulders squared, she moved past him

shoved an elbow in his ribs

shoved his handkerchief haphazardly into his breast pocket

slung the (*brown/leather*) strap of her purse over her shoulder

squatted and touched the spattering of dark red on the floor

squatted down to feed the fire another chunk of wood

standing abruptly to end the conversation

stood so close to him her chest nearly touched his

stood with his legs apart, in a warrior's stance

stopped at the door and looked back

stopped in front of her, his gaze running up and down her body

strode through a maze of linen and crystal set tables

struggled to a sitting position

swaggered into the (*bar/room*)

swung a leg over the corner of the (*desk/chair/table*)

taking a hearty sip

the muscular definition of his deltoids, his pectorals, his biceps

the old guy came panting across the yard to halt in front of her
took a long, cleansing breath

Fingers

💟~💟~💟~💟~💟~💟~💟~💟~💟~💟~💟~💟~💟~💟~💟~💟~💟~💟~💟

absently brushed his thumb back and forth over his chiseled jaw

absently traced the ball of his thumb across her cheek

bony, dirt crusted fingers

brushed at him with the backs of her chubby fingers

caressed (*his/her*) jaw

(*circled/closed*) (*his/her*) (*long, strong/hard and warm*) fingers on (*his/her*) wrist

closed his fingers around her wrist

cupped her chin in his hands

drummed the pads of her finger(*s*)/tips on the (*table/book*)

dug her fingernails into her palms

finger-fluffed her wind-blown hair

fingers (*dug/curled*) into her palms to keep from smacking the smirk off his face

fingers worked at the knotted muscles on her shoulders

gently brushed the dark curls back from his forehead

gently, tentatively she touched his dark hair

gently touched her face, his fingertips sliding over her cheekbone to her lips

hands large and calloused

he circled her wrist with his long fingers

he ran a hand through his thick hair and sighed

he touched her hair, just a light stroke

he took her hand in his and laced his fingers through hers

his fingers brushing over his bottom lip thoughtfully

his fingers digging into her (*arms/shoulders*)

his fingers encircling hers sent shivers up her arm

his fingers splayed downward along his groin, drawing attention to the impressive bulge

his fingers threaded through her hair

(*his/her*) fingers stroked through (*his/her*) hair

hooked his thumbs into his front pocket

lifted his free hand to stroke the skin of her neck where her jugular was

made a gun with his thumb and forefinger

massaged (*his/her*) temples briefly

one elegant, perfectly manicured hand

picked imaginary lint from her skirt

placed his right index finger across her lips

plunged her icy fingers into the pockets of her coat

pressing the pad of his thumb against her bottom lip, he forced her mouth open

raked his fingers through his hair as he glared at her

ran a finger over (*his/her*) jaw

ran her fingers through the shimmering strands of his hair

rolled the stem of his wineglass between his fingers

rubbed (*at his jaw/rubbed his jaw ruefully*)

slender, graceful fingers

smoothed a hand over her braids

snapped (*his/her*) her fingers

speared his hands through her hair

stroked a finger down her temple

stroked the corners of his mouth

stuck her face nose-to-nose with his and pressed a finger against his chest tapped a finger against her lips in a parody of thoughtfulness

tipped her chin up with his finger, wordlessly demanding she look at him

using a manicured finger she touched his square chin

Hands and Arms

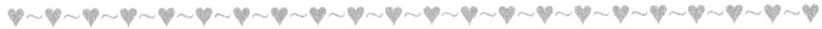

♥~♥~♥~♥~♥~♥~♥~♥~♥~♥~♥~♥~♥~♥~♥~♥~♥~♥~♥~♥

accepted a hearty hand shake

a hard hand gripped her wrist

approaching her with one hand held up like a traffic cop

arm curved around her to steady her

arm was around her, supporting her

arms bare and tanned beneath rolled up shirtsleeves

arms were brawny with hard-worked muscles

balled (*his/her*) fist

big workman's hands—broad across the palm with thick fingers

clapped him on the shoulder

clutched her purse hard against her breast

clutched her with tender strength

combed her mane of (*red/gold*) hair into a ponytail

cradled her face with his hands

cradled his chin in her hand and forced him to look up at her

(*crossed/folded*) (*his/her*) arms over (*his/her*) (*chest/breasts*)

curbed the urge to cover the spot he touched, trapping the heat that lingered there

dipped his hands into his pockets

dropping (*his/her*) hands (*he/she*) stepped back

extended one of his wide, capable hands

felt the firm steady grip as he steadied her

fists clenched as anger enveloped her

folded her arms under her breasts in a typical gesture of defense

folded her restless hands on the table

gently (*he/she*) (*touched/framed*) (*his/her*) face

gestured with (*his/her*) hands

grabbed the nape of her neck to force her gaze to his

grabbed the seatbelt with her other hand and pulled it around her

handed the empty glass back

hands (*clenched into fists/jammed into his pockets*)

hands like meat hooks

hand wrapped around her arm, turning her to him firmly

he dug his hands into the coil of her hair

held out (*his/her*) (*hand/an open hand*)

(*he/she*) firmly took hold of (*his/her*) elbow and led (*him/her*) to a chair

(*he/she*) (*held up/lifted*) (*his/her*) hand(s) in a gesture of surrender

her hand flew to her mouth to stop a startled gasp

her hands threaded through his soft hair

he winced, ran a hand through his hair

(*his/her*) hand closed into a white-knuckled fist

his hand landed in the middle of her back, anchoring her against him

his hand lingered, tracing the curve of her neck

his hands gentled on her, stroked up and down her arms

his hands gripped her shoulders and jerked her close

his hands moved across her body in the darkness

his massive hand halted her

holding the child's hand

instead of letting her go, he pulled her even closer to him

laughed and waved a hand

leaned forward, propping his elbows on his knees

lifted the binoculars to his eyes

lifted the glass to his lips and tipped it back

moved his large hands over her arms to her shoulders

noticed the tremor in (*his/her*) hands

one thin hand lifted toward (*him/her*)

picked her up, cradling her in his arms

picked up the drink and tossed it back with a single swallow

pinched the bridge of his nose

placing his palms on her shoulders

powerful arms rippled with movement

(*propped/put*) her hands on her hips

pumped his hand with enthusiasm

raked(*ing*) a hand through (*his/her*) hair, scraping the wet strands back from (*his/her*) (*face/forehead*)

ran a hand over (*him/her*), gently probing

reached for her hand, tucked it comfortably between his

reached out and moved the barrel of the shotgun away

reached up a hand and traced the hard angles of his face

rested his hand on the butt of his revolver

rubbed the bridge of his nose thoughtfully

rubbed the tense muscles in the back of his neck

(*rubbing/rubbed*) his hand over his (*face/jaw/neck/temples/forehead*)

rubbed the back of his neck with one pudgy hand

sat on the bed, tugging her down beside him

scrubbed a hand over his jaw

she pulled her arm from his grip

shielding her face from the deluge

shoved a hank of (*black*) hair in need of a trim out of his eyes

shoved both hands through his hair in agitation

shoving the heavy laden chip into his mouth

sighed, then slipped his hands into his pockets

stretched out (*his/her*) (*hand/arm/leg(s)*)

swept aside the (*items*)

tipped his champagne flute toward him in/a (*mock/ing*) salute

threw her hands in the air in a gesture full of exasperation

thrust a (*book/cup*) into her hands

thumb made slow, lazy circles on the back of her hand

tipped his hat back and looked down at her

wide calloused palms

wiped his mouth with the back of his hand

wrapped an arm around her shoulders, gave her a fatherly hug

wrapped (*his/her*) arms around (*him/her*)

Head Motions and Nods

♥~♥~♥~♥~♥~♥~♥~♥~♥~♥~♥~♥~♥~♥~♥~♥~♥~♥

gestured with his head to the other side of the room

had to tip her head up to look in his eyes

he groaned, then lowered his head

inclined (*his/her*) head in (*agreement/farewell*)

laid his cheek against the crown of her head

leaned (*back/her head*) against him

lifted her chin and narrowed a cold, hard look at him

lowered his head and kissed her

lowered his head to nuzzle the side of her face

lowered (*his/her*) head until their foreheads touched

nodded reluctantly

rubbed (*his/her*) cheek against (*him/her*)

shook her head, causing long skein of hair to ripple and sway

shook his head (*desperately/with a sharp jerk*)

spit out a wad of tobacco and wiped his mouth

stood, head bowed eyes hooded

studied the scuffed toes of (*his/her*) leather boots

taking a hearty sip

tilted her head back to better study his face

tilted her head back and looked into her eyes

tipped it back and downed a slug

took off his hat and nodded a greeting

Sitting, Standing, Walking, Running

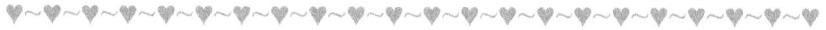

❤~❤~❤~❤~❤~❤~❤~❤~❤~❤~❤~❤~❤~❤~❤~❤~❤~❤~❤~❤

amble	beat feet	blunder in the dark
bolt	bound	bowlegged stride
bustle	casual manner	charge
crawl on all fours	creep, slip away	dart
dash	edge away	feline grace
flee	gait	hobble
hurry	hustle	jog
limp	loose limbed	lope
lurk	maneuver	meander
mosey	navigate	negotiate
pad	pert wiggle	plod
portly waddle	prowl	race
rush	sat prim/stick like	scamper
scoot	scurry	shuffle
skirt	slink away	sprint
storm out	stroll	strut
stumble	swagger	swoop
tear off	tip-toe	toddle
tread softly	trot	voluptuous sway
walk	wander aimlessly	weave

all too familiar stance of arrogant authority
crouched behind the hedge of bushes
eased down into a squat beside her
he towered over her
legs were trembling so badly she was afraid they wouldn't hold her
lengthened her stride to catch up

long legs churning up the distance in just a few strides

moved with the ease of a large jungle cat stalking its prey

moved with the grace and lightness of a vampire

pushed to (*his/her*) feet

rose and walked toward her all powerful grace and lean beauty

rose from the hard waiting room chair

sank into the desk chair

sat in a chair in a pool of lamp light

sauntered off, whistling a happy tune

settled his long, thin body into the seat

she walked with confidence

shifted his feet, awkward and ill at ease

shifted in his chair again

shifting around in his chair, as if the chair had suddenly become uncomfortable

sinking to one knee beside (*him/her*)

standing to the height of a giant

stepped back almost stumbling

stepped out of a chauffer-driven limo

stood as ruthless and proud as his reputation

strode across the distance with lazy ease

strode proudly and angrily inside

turned and strode away, his lithe muscled form moving with perfect grace

walked down the hallway with the gait of a predator

walked down the steps, stripping off his shirt casually, tossing it aside

walked toward her all powerful grace and lean beauty

whipped around to face her

Turns, Shrugs, Leaning

a shrug lifted her petite shoulders

bracing one hand on the window opening, he leaned down until they were eye-to-eye

careless shrug

(*he/she*) shrugged as though it didn't matter

leaned back and crossed her legs

leaned back, smoothed her tousled hair away from her forehead

leaned casually against the door frame

leaning back with false confidence as she crossed one leg over a knee

lifted a shoulder distinctly unimpressed

movements seemed slow and measured turning her toward him

she shrugged, fighting back the tears

she shrugged negligently

shrugged a meaty shoulder

turned in sudden anger and thumped her finger sharply against his chest

Body In Motion

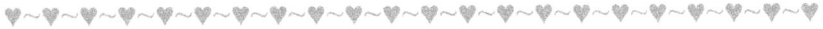

❤~❤~❤~❤~❤~❤~❤~❤~❤~❤~❤~❤~❤~❤~❤~❤~❤~❤~❤~❤

absently flexed cramped muscles

(*burst into/prowled around*) the room

came to his feet in an explosion of anger

caught her arm as she turned away from him

caught her by the arm, spinning her up against his chest

chest heaving laboriously

crossed his arms over his chest and glared down at her

cutting the distance between them with long, purposeful strides

did a formal little bow that made her feel like royalty

dipped (*his/her*) head, sighed wearily

dipped his shoulder and threw her over it

dismissed (*him/her*) with a negligent wave

drew (*his/her*) knees up, braced (*his/her*) forearms atop them, and let (*his/her*) hands dangle

dug in her heels and refused to back up

eased his bulk down

eased the pressure behind his zipper

ejecting himself from the chair

fell into a chair and reached for the phone

fluid, long-legged gait of a dangerous predator

folded her hands primly in front of her

glanced back out the window

grabbed his jeans, jamming first one leg and then the other in

grabbed his Stetson and sheepskin coat from the antler rack

gripped her shoulders and jerked her closer

he crossed his arms, the muscles bunching beneath the thick cotton of his shirt

heaved his considerable bulk out of his high-backed leather chair

he hugged her, rubbing his cheek against the top of her head

held up both hands in a classic gesture of innocence

helped her to her feet

he moved like a panther, watching, stalking, waiting

(*he/she*) came crawling across the bed to (*him/her*)

(*he/she*) cocked (*his/her*) hip against (*item*)

(*he/she*) had a slow seductive walk

(*he/she*) (*moved close/in closer*) to look

(*he/she*) reluctantly pushed away from the counter

(*he/she*) shuffled down a short hallway

(*he/she*) (*spun/pushing past*) (*him/her*)

(*he/she*) tilted (*his/her*) chair back

(*he/she*) walked with confidence

(*he/she*) watched (*him/her*) pace, appreciating the way (*he/she*) moved

he sighed and (*tucked/hugged*) heroine a little tighter

he watched her slender back retreat

his back muscles were a masterpiece of movement under his shirt

hitched at his pants

hooked an ankle over his knee

kneeling next to (*him/her*)

let out a slow controlled breath

lifting her up until her feet dangled helplessly above the ground

limped to a chair and eased into it

long, thoroughbred legs sashaying under the sexy silk skirt

looked down into the coffee cup in (*his/her*) hand

mopped the sweat from (*his/her*) forehead

one elbow resting casually over the arm of the chair

paced the den wringing her hands as tears streamed from her eyes

picked her up, threw her over his shoulder in a fireman's hold

propped arms on the table (*he/she*) was sitting at

pulled open the door and sailed through it with queenly grace

pushed away from the truck and came toward (*him/her*)

reached around and dragged her up against his hard body

removed (*his/her*) clothing with thoughtful measured movements

rested his hip on the side of the car and crossed his arms over his chest

retraced her steps to him with a sexy swagger

scooped her into his arms

shaded (*his/her*) eyes against the brilliance of the rising sun

shrugged and spread his hands to indicate helplessness

shrugged a slow roll of one massive shoulder

silence fell as (*he/she*) stuck (*his/her*) hands in (*his/her*) pockets and said nothing

sinking to one knee beside (*him/her*)

skirt pulled high up on her (*legs/thighs*) when she sat

slammed the full liquor bottle on the counter

slid into (*his/her*) arms

snuggling in (*deep, deeper/tighter*)

spread (*his/her*) feet further apart and stuck the tips of (*his/her*) fingers into (*his/her*) back pockets

spun on her clunky heeled boots and sauntered away

squared her shoulders

staggered through the door

stalked to the bedroom and slammed the door

stood nose-to-nose

stretched (*his/her*) long, jean-clad legs out in front of (*him/her*) and picked up (*his/her*) cooling coffee

straightened with unhurried grace

strolled around (*his/her*) bedroom

taking the stairs two at a time

the mattress gave beneath his weight, rolling her gently against his thigh

the mere idea stopped (*him/her*) cold

they stood nose to nose

threw open the door and stepped aside

thrust the (*cup/book/papers*) into her hands

tipped his chin back indicating the vague direction of the club

took a deliberate step closer

took one meaningful step forward

turned on his heel and snapped out commands like a general on the battlefield

turned toward the door, then turned back

walking with the grace of a fairy princess

watched her walk down the hall, enjoying the gentle sway of hips and stride of long, sexy legs

whirled her around, spinning her out to the end of his fingertips and then flicked her back

with a snap of his strong wrist, he spun her away from him and pulled her back again

with a toss of her head

Dancing

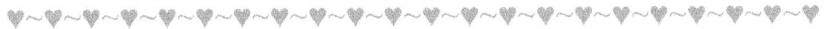

all around her bodies moved and slid against her

all but purring she leaned into him

a slow ballad that paired up the sweaty bodies

anchored her to him with a possessiveness that stunned

as quickly as his body heat disappeared, it was back

delicious sensation shot through her entire body

drawing her into his arms

drew her politely into his arms and swayed to the music (*of the ballad/blasting around them*)

faster and faster the music played, driving her higher and higher

fortunately she could work dancing as a form of seduction

glut of bodies grinding to the beat with (*surreal/carnal*) beauty

he found a place in the middle of the swaying couples

he half growled, half laughed and pulled her even closer

he laughed and twirled her away from him again, then gathered her close once more

he led her quickly off the dance floor and toward the back exit of the club

he lifted her against him as he spun around the room, her feet barely skimming the floor

he maneuvered her into the thick of the crowd of dancers

her boots kicking up sawdust as she danced and had the time of her life

he whirled her around, spinning her out to the end of his fingertips and then flicking her back

his arms snaked around her waist, pulling her tight

his body was flexible steel against hers

his hand landed in the middle of her back, anchoring her
sinfully against him

instead of letting her go, he pulled her even closer to him

instinctively following the subtle signals of his body as he led
her around (*the dance floor*)

music blasted from multiple speakers

music throbbed in time with the pulsing desire between her
thighs

she danced as she went about her task, her hips moving

she gasped as he spun her around in a fast (*jive*) step

she let him lead her to the dance floor

she melted against him, threading her fingers in his hair

she plastered herself to him from shoulder to knee

sighed in delight and as he swayed them back and forth

slid his arms around her waist and brought her up against his
tuxedo jacket

swayed in sinuous rhythm to the song

(*swayed/danced/moved*) like sensual energy

sweaty bodies bumping into her

the club was packed, gyrating bodies all around (*her, them*)

the dance floor was hot and crowded

the leaden beat off a bass guitar pulsed through her head

the music was earthy, raw

the song changed tempo and a driving beat pounded through
his body into hers

with a snap of his strong wrist, he spun her away from him and
pulled her back again

wrapped in his arms, her head rested on his shoulder

Complexion

Skin Color

alabaster	albino	apple blossom
black	blush	brown
café au lait	café noir	caramel
Caucasian	chalky	charcoal
chestnut	china doll	china silk
cinnamon	coal	cocoa
cream	dusky	ebony
eggshell	fair	ginger
golden	honey	ivory
lily-white	magnolia	midnight
milky	molasses	nut-brown
olive	peach	pink
pitch	sandalwood	sepia
tar	teakwood	sun-browned
strawberries and cream		

Reddish

bloom	blush	floridness
glow	high color	inflammation
rosiness	rubenesque	ruddiness

Skin Types

acned/zits	age spots	alligator
apple-cheeked	blanched	blemished
cadaverous	chalky	cratered
cyanotic	dermatitis	doughy
downy	eczema	florid
flush	freckled	glowing
greasy	jaundiced	leathery
livid	molted	pale
pallid	pasty	pitted
pizza-faced	pocked	pustuled
razor-burned/rosy	ruddy	sallow
sandpaper	scarred	scrubbed
splotchy	sunburned	swarthy
wan	warty	waxy
wheat	weather-beaten	withered

Sunburned

bronzed	brown/browned	burned
crimson	lobster	sunburned/sunburnt
tan/tanned	toasted	

Additional

fair	light	pale
paleface	tow-head	

Eyes

Expression

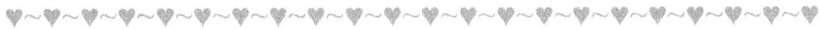

admiring gaze	attentive	anxiousness
blink	blinked owlishly	burned
bright	crinkle mirthfully	dance/and sparkle
dangerous	dark	deep
defiant	determination	frigid stare
furtive look	fury	gawk
gaze/glance	glare	gleamed
glower	haunted eyes	leer/leer nastily
lifted	monstrous glare	mysterious
observe	ogle	peek
probing eyes	regard	rolled her eyes
scorching look	scowl	scrutiny
sensual	sharpened	shoot daggers
smoldered	sparkle	squint
stare	stared back at	study acutely
view	warming	watch
watchful	wide with alarm	wink
wounded look		

a flat lack of emotion in his eyes

a long, silent, sizing up moment

mixture of interest and compassion filling her (*turquoise/blue*) eyes a suggestive look over her shoulder

a (*threatening stare/violent light in his dark eyes*)

a (*wicked/sensual/determined*) gleam lit (*his/her*) eyes

amused gleam in (*his/her*) eyes was breathtaking

as their gazes locked, there was a moment of sizzling awareness

(*blue/green*) eyes snapping in (*challenge/defiance/warning*)

(*blue/gray*) eyes (*filled with mischief/twinkling in fun*)

blue eyes, serious and brooding

brimmed with (*joy/tears*)

close set eyes, blazing red

closed (*his/her*) eyes, took a deep breath

closed (*his/her*) eyes briefly

closed (*his/her*) eyes tightly and swallowed

closing her eyes, she drew in a slow, calming breath

cold (*fury/purpose*) glittered in (*his/her*) eyes

continued to study him with eyes as sharp and savvy as his own

could cut a (*woman/man*) off at the knees with just a glance

crinkled with laughter

crystal-blue gaze glowed with warm curiosity and intelligence

curtained with heavy, dark lashes

damp with tears of joy

dark centers of his eyes dilated until she thought she would melt

dark, (*earnest eyes/mystical gaze*)

dark shadows filled (*his/her*) once (*happy/joyous*) gaze

dark with pain

defiance flashed through (*his/her*) eyes

exotic quality to her almond-shaped eyes

expression filled with (*anxiousness/uneasy worry*)

expression stamped with male arrogance and command

eyed skeptically

eyes (*alive with anger/icy cold/predatory/full of pain*)

eyes (*blazed/flared/smoldered*) with unspoken desire

eyes blazed (*murderously/with cold purpose/with mischief*)

eyes (*bright/alive*) with (*mischief/anger/pain*)

eyes (*bulged, narrowed/burned/gleamed/mocked*)

eyes burned bright with a rabid fervor

eyes (*danced/sparkled/studied acutely*)

eyes danced with the beginning of a smile

eyes deep, dark and mysterious as they gazed into (*his/hers*)

eyes deep pools of (*black/dark*) savagery

eyes filled with anxiousness

eyes flickered with rage

eyes (*full of/filled with*) (*intelligence/mockery/mischief/ sexuality*)

(*eyes/gaze*) hard, cold, like the freezing wind

(*eyes/gazes*) (*locked/glittered with defiance*)

(*eyes/gaze*) quiet, solemn, apologetic

eyes huge and bright

eyes icy and filled with a promise of retribution

eyes looked at (*him/her*) with mad desperation

eyes narrowed at the challenge in his voice

eyes narrowed with disgust

eyes predatory and liquid hot

eyes sharpened at the information

eyes shining with excitement

eyes snaring hers and holding them against her will

eyes, stark and black as night filled with bitterness

eyes that could hypnotize with a glance

eyes that flashed with shimmering gold sparks

eyes that had seen more than (*he/she*) could ever imagine

eyes that smiled at him, that offered so much

eyes took (*his/her*) measure

eyes were cool, cynical as they watched (*him/her*)

eyes were dark, tortured

eyes were molten with defiance

eyes widened innocently

filled with warm intelligence and vitality

flames of anger simmered in her eyes

flicked him an amused look from beneath her lashes

flashing him an angry look

(*flickered/filled*) with (*hot fury/rage/angry confusion*)

for one (*humming/vibrant*) minute they stared at each other

full of (*assessment/male arrogance/understanding*)

gave (*him/her*) an insulting once-over

gaze settled on that sassy mouth of hers

gazed at him with undisguised concern

genuine (*compassion/relief/remorse*) in her eyes

glanced over (*his/her*) shoulder

gleamed with laughter

gleam in his eyes turned (*carnal/wicked*)

glinted, shone with pleasure

glittered with lust

gray eyes dark and thunderous

grew dark and sultry with (*pleasure/promise/wicked intent*)

hated knowing he had put that look of (*contempt/fear/anger*) in her lovely eyes hated the (*trapped/wounded*) animal look in (*his/her*) eyes

haunting shadows flashed in (*his/her*) gaze

he tipped her face up forcing her to see the truth in his eyes

(*he/she*) had the most incredible eyes (*he'd/she'd*) ever seen

(*he/she*) kept (*his/her*) eyes on the floor

(*he/she*) stared back (*his/her*) expression thoughtful

(*he/she*) was watching (*him/her*) silently, calculating

heavy-lidded stare

held the (*boy's/girl's*) eyes with mesmerizing force

her eyes filled with pain and tears broke his heart

her eyes gleamed with laughter

his gaze made her body tingle in a foreign and wicked way

his gaze starkly possessive

(*his/her*) expression (*becoming darker/fierce/furious*)

(*his/her*) eyes could carve a (*man/woman*) to pieces at ten paces

(*his/her*) eyes (*unwavering/doubtful*)

(*his/her*) eyes flared wide

(*his/her*) gaze burned her with intelligence and unholy power

(*his/her*) gaze on the horizon

(*his/her*) gaze warming (*him/her*), touching (*him/her*)

(*his/her*) narrow gaze sharpened on (*his/her*) face, watched (*him/her*) expectantly

(*his/her*) prolonged stare sent a rush of desire coiling through (*him/her*)

(*his/her*) wild blue eyes darkened just a bit

hungry, predatory look in his eyes

if looks could kill she'd need a permit for those eyes

intensity of his dark gaze seemed to suck the air out of her lungs

intriguing eyes that hinted at a heart full of secrets

it was his eyes that got to her, (*greenish/brown*) with lashes long and curved

keep-your-mouth-shut look

large, expressive eyes were luminous and mischievous

large, heavily-lined eyes that looked mysterious and sensual

(*laser blue/gray/brown*) eyes met hers, direct and probing

long-lashed, (*black/brown/blue*) eyes

long, searching look

looked him in the eye, marshaling all her defenses

looked up at him with those trusting (*blue/green*) eyes

met (*his/her*) eyes without (*apology/remorse*)

misty, cloudy with sadness

no reprieve or mercy in his (*eyes/gaze*)

nonchalantly his (*golden/sensual*) gaze dropped to her lips

nonchalantly studied the nails on one hand

opened (*his/her*) eyes to see fury reflected in (*his/hers*)

pupils dilated and dark rimmed in an eerie (*topaz/green*)

quiet strength in (*his/her*) eyes

raw sexual heat in his gaze

read understanding in (*his/her*) deep, (*blue/green/color*) eyes

reddened from hours of weeping

regard (*critically/curiously*)

rolled (*his/her*) eyes (*mockingly/and groaned*)

saw the look of (*devilment/irritation*) in (*his/her*) eyes

shadowed with (*bitterness/worry/a hint of anger*)

she had eyes that made men forget to breathe

(*shining/glinting*) with pleasure

smiled at the temper smoldering in (*his/her*) eyes

spared a glance at the blatant invitation

sparkling, (*dark/intense*) eyes held both humor and intelligence

squinting against the harsh sunlight

stared at (*him/her*) with harsh contempt

studied (*him/her*) with (*his/her*) solemn eyes

surprised by the vicious flash of heat in (*his/her*) eyes

tears came and this time she didn't stop them

the cold glitter (*in/of*) (*his/her*) gaze

the hurt that surrounded them in (*his/her* eyes)

the seductive gleam in his storm-filled gaze threatened to make
a liar of her

those incredible eyes were narrowed in concentration

thoughtful and expressive

through the deepening twilight she could see the stormy
tension in his eyes

too full of life's hard knocks

tried to keep her eyes locked on his face, but they drifted over
his body anyway

watched as (*his/her*) eyes darkened

watched the battle that raged in (*his/her*) eyes

wicked eyes hidden behind black shades

worry darkening the color of (*his/her*) expression

Movement

♥~♥~♥~♥~♥~♥~♥~♥~♥~♥~♥~♥~♥~♥~♥~♥~♥~♥~♥~♥

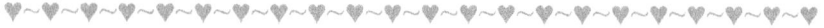

a mocking glance

big, (*hazel/brown/blue*) eyes questioning

blinked the spray of rain from his eyes

blinked with surprise

eyes darted from one to the other, panicked, pleading

eyes followed her every move

eyes seemed to swirl like phantom mists

eyes serious and brooding

eyes wide and wild with shock

felt (*his/her*) gaze, as a physical blow

forced (*his/her*) eyes open

gave him a (*pointed look/wink*) and walked off

gaze sliding casually down her body before rising to meet hers again

gazed out over the ancient hills

glanced up from beneath her lashes

her gaze skated over his bare chest, then lower

her heavy eyelashes fluttered just before she lifted them

(*his/her*) eyes captured (*his/hers*) and did not let go

(*his/her*) eyes dancing

lifted his (*beady/tiny*) eyes

looked at him with big, tired, sad eyes

narrowed a cold look at (*him/her*)

narrowed (*eyes/gaze*) with promised retribution

narrowed with (*contempt/disdain/disgust/suspicion*)

narrowing eyes the color of (*electric blue/slate gray/green*)

she flicked him an amused look from (*beneath/under*) her lashes

slow, appraising glance

slowly (*lifted/lowered*) (*his/her*) gaze

stared adoringly at the puppy

stared at (*him/her*) gravely

stared back at (*him/her*) broodingly

stared down at her with smoldering intensity

stared down at (*his/her*) own reflection in (*his/her*) sunglasses

staring furiously down at her surprised face

the image of his wink stayed with her long after he was gone

lacy fringe of her lashes lifted

thick-lashed, brown eyes were dark-shadowed

watched (*him/her*) over the rim of (*his/her*) (*coffee/beer*)

when she blinked, her (*long/full/lush*) lashes lightly caressed (*high/regal*) cheekbones

Type and Shape

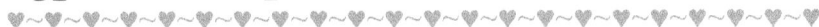

almond	banjo	beady
bug	bulging	bullish
button	close-set	crescent
cross-eyed	deep-set	dew drop
feline	fish	glassy
hooded	luminous	oriental
owlish	pea	saucer
shark-like	slanty	slits
spaniel	squinty	sunken
wide-set		

Additional Descriptions

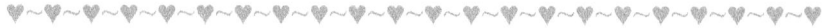

♥~♥~♥~♥~♥~♥~♥~♥~♥~♥~♥~♥~♥~♥~♥~♥~♥~♥~♥

a violent light in his dark eyes

a wicked gleam came into his eyes

(*blue*) eyes had cooled, sharpened and gone deadly serious

caught in the trap of her blue eyes like a fly in a spider's web

confusion in her wide, (*blue*) eyes

crow's-feet at the corners of his eyes

eyes darkened with a ruthless determination

eyes blazing with anger and hate

eyes burned bright with a rabid fervor

eyes dark and frightened in the pale frame of her face

eyes narrowed, becoming dark slits of pure fury

eyes narrowed, flat and dark at the insult

eyes that could scramble the senses of a less weary (*man/woman*)

eyes were cold and hard with bitterness

felt the intimate probe of (*his/her*) eyes

he stared down at her and she could feel the heat sizzling in his (*color*) eyes

her eyelashes made dark crescents on her suntanned cheeks

(*his/her*) eyes flared in the darkness as (*he/she*) closed the distance between (*him/her*)

his eyes were hard and inscrutable

huge with fatigue

in (*his/her*) eyes lay the wisdom of the ages

in his gaze she saw the fierce power of a good, honest man

intense (*eyes/gaze*) that for a moment held (*him/her*) prisoner

lifted one (*black/dark)*) brow in an elegant gesture of disdain

long, (*coal/black*) lashes fluttered

narrowed (*his/her*) eyes gauging whether (*he/she*) was telling the truth

(*old/dark/haunted*) eyes were blank and unseeing

one hideously white, blind eye

pale, deep-set eyes

snakelike, unblinking eyes

those incredible eyes of (*his/hers*) knocked (*him/her*) for a loop

Create Your Own Tags!!!

Eye Color

Blue and Green

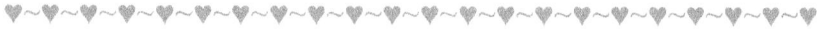

♥~♥~♥~♥~♥~♥~♥~♥~♥~♥~♥~♥~♥~♥~♥~♥~♥

apple-green	azure	baby-blue
blueberry	bottle green	bittersweet
celestial blue	cobalt	cornflower
denim	dove gray	electric blue
emerald	grape	holly green
hyacinth	ice	indigo
iris	jade	jungle
lagoon blue	lapis lazuli	larkspur
lavender	lightning	lilac
midnight-blue	misty-blue	morning glory
moss	nightshade	Nordic blue
olive-green	passionflower	peacock blue
periwinkle	plum	powder-blue
rainforest green	royal purple	sapphire
sea	sea green	sea smoke
sky-blue	slate	smoke
smoked glass	snow-shadow	star
steel	storm	teal
twilight	violet	Virginia bluebell
wild lupine	wisteria blue	

Dark

♥~♥

acorn	autumn leaf	biscuit
bronze	burnt almond	camel
congo	dun	dusky
earth	ebony	elk
fawn	fox	gunmetal
hawk brown	hazel	honey
kelp	leather	lentil
mahogany	mink	Mississippi
molasses	mud	nut-brown
obsidian	olive	otter
raisin	raven	russet
sandy	seaweed	soot
sorrel	sparrow	tarnished penny
taupe	tawny	umber

Description of Eye Color

♥~♥

a faint tinge of black and blue next to one of her eyes

a ring of gold overlaid on icy (*sky blue/gray*)

big, (*blue/azure*) eyes mirroring the color of the sky

(*black/green*), widely spaced

(*brown/green*) eyes tinged with amber that slanted up like a cat

clear, pure green

dark as sin, fringed with thick charcoal lashes

(*dark-blue/slate gray*) eyes that were vibrant and direct

dark eyes as shiny and opaque as wet slate

dark eyes framed by thick, ebony lashes

doe (*brown/blue*) eyes

drowsy, whiskey colored eyes

enigmatic, tiger-gold eyes

evenly spaced, light (*brown/blue*)

eyes (*dark gray/blue-gray*) as a winter storm

eyes like a winter sky reflected in chips of ice

fire and ice clashing in discord

fire and intelligence burned deep in her (*dark/brown*) eyes

hard, black unforgiving eyes

(*hazel-green/blue-gray*) eyes filled with a brilliant vitality

his eyes a lazy shade of blue, seemed to burn right into her

intense, pale (*gray/green*) eyes

pale (*blue/green*) gaze glowed faintly, even in the dark

she had never seen such eyes, they were bottomless, and as clear as...

(*silvery/cat-like/startling/somber brown/gray*) eyes

slumberous and (*blue/brown*)

summer-sky eyes full of curiosity and mischief

the color like (*semi-sweet chocolate/brown sugar/cinnamon*)

the pale color reminded him of fine whiskey

there was un unspoken challenge in the depths of (*his/her*) midnight blue eyes

tobacco-brown eyes were lit with an inner fire

whiskey eyes shimmered with golden depths and framed by thick, dark lashes

whiskey eyes that stretched long and exotic beneath dramatic dark brows

(*wide/liquid*), (*dark/brown*) eyes

Hair

Color

♥~♥

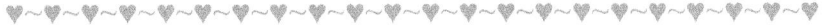

acorn	alabaster	ash
ash blonde	auburn	black
bleached	bleached-blond	blond/blonde
blue-gray	brown	bottle blond
brunette	buckskin	burnt almond
café au lait	caramel	chestnut
chocolate	cinnamon	coal black
cocoa	coffee	copper
fair-haired	fawn	fiery
flaming	flaxen	flint
fox	golden	gray
grizzled	henna	honey
ivory	jet black	light-haired
magnolia	maple-sugar	mocha
nut-brown	natural blond	nutmeg
peroxide blonde	platinum blonde	polished wood
premature gray	raven	russet
rust	sable	salt and pepper
sandalwood	sandy-haired	silver
smoke	snowy	straw
strawberry blonde	tarnished sunset	tawny
technicolor	titian	tow-head
washed-out	white	yellow-haired

Styles

afro	bangs	beehive
beetle cut	bob	bouffant
boyish bob	braids	brushed back
bun	chignon	coiled
corkscrew curls	cornrows	crew cut
dreadlocks	ducktail	elf-locks
fade	feather-cut	fishbone braid
flat-top	flip	French braid
man bun	Mohawk	pageboy
pigtails	pixie	poodle cut
punk	receding hair line	rooster mane
sculptured	shag	shock
skinhead	spikes	spit curl
tail	topknot	wedge
widow's peak		

Textures

baby fine	billowing	bird's nest
bouncy	bristly	bushy
coarse	corn-silk	crinkly
dollish	down	downy
eider	fleecy	flowing
flyaway	frazzled	frizzy
fuzzy	greasy	kinky
knotted	lacquered	listless

Hair

lustrous	luxurious	matted
nappy	oily	rat's nest
rigid	ropey	satiny
shaggy	silky	snarled
spiky	stringy	thatched
wiry	wispy	wooly

Voice

Used with Quotes

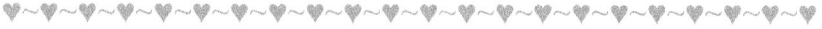

added	asked	barked
began	bellowed	breathed
buzzed	disclosed	divulged
exclaimed	growled	hissed
hinted	hummed	insinuated
interrupted	intimated	mumbled
murmur	muttered	queried
replied	resumed	revealed
rumored	rustled	said
screamed	shrieked	sighed
snapped	snarled	sneered
stammered	whispered	wondered

Types

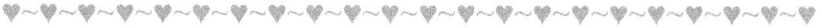

accent	angry	breathy
cackling	calm	clearing throat
cracking voice	crying	deep
disguised	distinct	excited
familiar	laughter	lisp
loud	nasal	normal
ragged/rough	rapid	raspy
slow	slurred	soft
stutter	whispered	

Tones: Anger

♥~♥~♥~♥~♥~♥~♥~♥~♥~♥~♥~♥~♥~♥~♥~♥~♥~♥~♥~

acidly	barbed	bitterly
bluntly	boldly	brazenly
caustically	coldly	crudely
defensively	fiercely	frigidly
fume	furiously	gruffly
harsh	haughtily	(*he/she*) said
hiss	hotly	icily
in a huff	incredulously	indignantly
maliciously	moodily	ruthlessly
sarcastically	sardonically	savagely
self-righteously	sharply	sourly
spitefully	stubbornly	tart
testily	venomously	

Tones: Fear

♥~♥~♥~♥~♥~♥~♥~♥~♥~♥~♥~♥~♥~♥~♥~♥~♥~♥~♥~

bawl	breaks	cry out
groan	high and hysterical	howl
lowers to a childish whisper		moan
maniacal laugh	screams	shriek
shrill with terror	sob	strangled cry
wail	whimper	

95

Exclamations

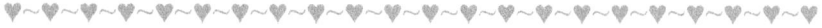

♥~♥~♥~♥~♥~♥~♥~♥~♥~♥~♥~♥~♥~♥~♥~♥~♥~♥~♥~♥

A
ack	(ah/aha/ahh)	ahem
abso-fucking-lutely	argh	aw/aw shucks
aye	atta boy	atta girl

B
bada bing	bada bing, bada boom	
(bah/blah)	bite me	blah blah blah
bless our heart	bloody hell	blow me
boo-hoo	boo-ya/booyah	

C
(capeesh/capiche/capisce)	caramba
cha-ching	correctamundo
(crimenetly/criminently/criminetly)	criminy
cripes	cute as a button

D
d'oh	dad burn	dadgum
dadgummit	(dag/dagnabbit/dagnabit/dagnammit)	
(damme/damn/dayum)		
(damnit/damn it/dammit)		dammit to hell
damn and blast	damn straight	damn your eyes
damn your hide	dang/dang it	darn
(dang tootin'/tooting)	(darn tootin'/durn tootin)	
(dear me/dearie me/deary me)		diddums
doggone		dy-no-mite

E

easy does it	eat my dust	eat my shorts
eat shit	eaw	ecky thump
ee	eek	eep
eew	eff all	egad
egads	eh	en garde

F

fa shizzle	fiddledeedee	fiddlefart
fiddlesticks	fie	fire in the hole
fit to be tied	fixin to	fo/fo' shizzle
fo shizzle my nizzle	foggetaboutit	

G

gadzooks	get outta here	giddap
gidday	giddy up/yup	God willing
goddammit	goddamn	goddamnit
goddang	goldarn	goldarnit
goldurn	goldurnit	good God
good going	good golly	good gracious
good gravy	good grief	good heavens
good job	good Lord	good luck
good morning	good morrow	good now
good riddance	good show	good-by/goodbye
goodie	goodness gracious	
goodness gracious me		goodness me

H

hardy har har	harrumph	harumph
hell	hell and tommy	hell no/Hell no
hell or high water	hell's bells	hell's teeth
hella	hissy fit	(hm/hmm/hmmm)

hmph   (ho hum/ho-hum)   holy cow
holy crap   holy crap on a cracker
holy cricket(s)   holy fuck   holy guacamole
(holy kamoley/kamoly)   holy mackerel
(holy moley/moly)   holy Moses   Holy Mother
Holy Mother of God   holy shit   holy smoke
holy Toledo   hoorah   horse hockey
horsefeathers

J
Jeebus   jeez   jeez Louise
Jeezum Crow   Jesus   Jesus Christ
Jesus H. Christ   Jesus Harold Christ   Judas Priest
jumping Jehoshaphat   jumping Jesus
jumpity

K
kazaam   kerblam   kerboom
kerchoo   kerplop   kerplunk
kerpow   kersplat

L
la-di-da   lackaday   (lah-de-dah/lah-di-dah)
like to

M
mmhm   mmhmm   mmkay
mmm   my arse   my ass
my bad   my eye   my foot
my giddy aunt   my God   my goodness
my Lord   my my   my pleasure
my sainted aunt   my sainted uncle   my word

O

oh	oh boy	oh dear
oh God	Oh-oh	oh man
oh my	oh my days	oh my God
oh my Goddess	oh my goodness gracious	
oh my heck	oh my hell	oh my Lord
oh my stars	oh no	oh well
oh-oh	ohmigod	(oooh/ooooh)
oops	(oopsie/oopsy)	oorah

S

sheesh	Shh

T

ta-da	tsk	tsk-tsk

U

ugh	uh	(uh uh/uh huh/uh-huh)
uh-oh	(uh uh/uh-uh)	uh-oh, Spaghetti-O
uhh	u-huh	ugh
uh	uh huh	(uh oh/uh-oh)
um	unh-uh	

W

well done	well said	well, I never
(well/well,well)	whoa	whaddayaknow
whaddayamean	whaddayasay	whaddayathink
whaddayawant	whoah	whoo
whoomp	whoopee	

(whoopee do/whoopee-do/whoopee-doo)

(woops/whoops)	(whoops-a-daisy/whoopsadaisy)	
(whoopsy/whoopsy-daisy)		why/wuzzup

Y

yee-haw/yeehaw	yeees	yeeha
yeek	yeep	yeesh
yeh	yeow	yeowch
yes	yes way	yes'm
yessir	yessiree/yessirree	you betcha
you don't say	yoo hoo	yikes
yipe	yipes	(yippee/yippie)
yippee skippy	yippie ki-yay	yo
yeh	yes	yes way
yes'm	yessir	(yessiree/yessirree)
yee-haw	(yea/yeah)	yeah right
yeah, no	yecch	

Z
'zactly

Manners of Speech

a bittersweet crest of emotion filled (*his/her*) voice
a deep slightly aggravated sigh
a full-throated, wicked, carnal sound of hunger
a knife couldn't have been sharper than (*his/her*) voice
a low voice that reverberated through her like a lingering caress
anger thickening (*his/her*) voice
a note of triumph in his voice
a soft moan of pleasure and desire
a (*smooth, dark, old voice/dark, strangely accented voice*)
a thin thread of mania in (*his/her*) voice
an edge of excitement to (*his/her*) voice

began to chant in (*his/her*) ancient language

bit back a soft appreciative moan

chuckled mockingly

could hear (*his/her*) quiet voice, murmuring words of comfort

deceptively soft, smooth as he started toward her

deep masculine baritone murmuring in her ear

deep, smoothly accented voice that rumbled like thunder

deep voice was mesmerizing and filled with promise

deeply male, and touched with exasperation and concern

disgust (*filled/lined*) his voice

drawled, his voice sending vibrations deep into the core of her body

edge of command in his voice

even and infinitely patient

even, authoritative and no nonsense

excitement throbbed in his voice

filled with rolling R's and softly dropped G's

French, aristocratic and deep

Georgia peaches and cream accent

(*he/she*) suddenly lost (*his/her*) power of speech

(*he/she*) cleared (*his/her*) throat and continued

he spoke in an agonized whisper that tore at her heart

heard the hint of teasing in (*his/her*) voice

her voice vibrating with (*feeling/desperation*)

her words faded to a whisper

high edge of fear colored (*his/her*) voice

his (*firm no-nonsense voice/deep-booming voice*)

(*his/her*) tone low and purring

Rebecca Andrews

(*his/her*) voice held (*a heavy, ancient Celtic accent/a charming French lilt*)

(*his/her*) voice held no mercy, no passion

(*his/her*) voice, like long vowels dipped in (*melted/creamy*) chocolate

(*his/her*) voice (*shook, broke/hitch in*) (*his/her*) voice

(*his/her*) voice (*velvet, southern drawl/a soft, slow accent/rich Irish Cream/cultured/smoky/velvety*)

(*his/her*) voice was (*cold/flat/furious/shook with strain*)

(*his/her*) voice was a velvet soft, rasp of pleasure

his voice (*a growl of caged fury/edge of impatience/low, brutal*)

his voice a low vibration that shivered through her soul

his voice an aching rasp that curled through her on a wave of heat

his voice (*a soft growl/husky, hoarse/low disturbing, sexy/ whiskey rough/unbearably sexy*)

his voice (*firm no-nonsense/deep-booming*)

his voice, like his dark hair, was smooth and oily

his voice low, masculine and oh so sure of himself

his voice made her want to lean closer and revel in the sensuous baritone

his voice rumbled out of the darkness startling her

his voice slipped over her like crushed velvet

his voice strained, taut with need

his voice was (*cold and steady as stone/firm/rough hewn/ brisk/business like*)

(*his/her*) words chilled (*him/her*) to the bone

(*his/her*) words were simply spoken and right to the point

his words were soft, buffeting her skin, raising a shiver

his words were smooth, low and disarming

his words wound like silken threads around her heart

kept his (*voice calm/his tone gentle*)

let out a (*careful/controlled*) breath

lifeless tone to (*his/her*) voice

liked the cadence of her voice

lost in the haunted sorrow of (*his/her*) voice

lowered his voice to a silky softness

murder swirled in the dark cadence of his voice

murmured (*in that hypnotizing voice of his/mocking drawl*)

muttered something unintelligible under her breath

rasped (*his/her*) name with heated passion

rich with a thick lilting accent

rough, deep, filled with arrogant demand

said (*his/her*) name (*softly/with soft menace*)

savagery in his voice

she asked with saccharine sweetness and innocence

she huffed and muttered

she laughed, a husky draft of amusement

she said with a breeziness he recognized as dismissal

silky menace of (*his/her*) tone

silvery laughter tinkling on the night breeze

sinfully rich, melodious voice that made her toes curl

slightly raspy voice with a burred inflection

smooth southern drawl, like black velvet in the darkness

smooth southern drawl that rolled off (*his/her*) tongue

soft and filled with caution

soft moan of pleasure and desire

speech peppered with French expressions

spoke in a voice so serene it surprised even her

spoke the words in a breathy rush

spoke with a quiet intensity that brought her eyes around to meet his

strong, confident, tantalizingly sweet

taunted in a deep resonate tone that went down her spine like warm velvet

the cadence of his low, rough voice sent an odd jolt to the pit of her belly

the desperate voice came out of its own accord

the lazy sensuality of his voice called to her

the sound of his own voice woke him

the (*man/woman*) spoke slow and easy with a (*Texan/Southern/other*) accent

there was such impeccable surety in his voice

thick with an exotic accent

though the words were softly spoken there was an underlying steel to them

throaty, unique voice, low, intimate and mocking

tight note in his voice hinted at concern

tone held an air of unequivocal authority

tone was classic male mockery

unaware of the way her voice softened as she reached for...

voice caught in her throat on a horrified whisper

voice (*cold and certain/flat and careful*)

voice deep and sinfully rich

voice dripped southern debutante

voice dropped a purposeful octave

voice held (*an unusual edge/a teasing lightness*)

voice like aged whiskey

Voice

voice like thick molasses covered in dark chocolate

voice low and beautifully modulated

voice (*low, brutal/challenging/thick with insinuation*)

voice rumbled like distant thunder

voice sounded robotic and stripped of emotion

voice (*throbbed with power/vibrated with dark desire*)

voice vibrated through her in an erotic wave

voice was light, sweet and liquidly southern

voice was rough and close as it whispered across her face

voice was torn, rough, thick

warm and lush, his voice stroked her senses

whiskey smooth and maddeningly sexy

whispered against the soft silk of her hair

whispered wearily

whispery voice that feathered along his nerve endings

words had been quietly spoken

Negative Expressions

a rough, unbelieving laugh

angry outburst stopped her cold

bitter (*mockery/regret*) filled her voice

chilly, precise, dry, little voice

chuckled mockingly

cold as death

disgust lined his voice/dripping with spite

had a high and effeminate voice

her voice took on a sweetness that made him grind his clenched jaw

105

laughed brutally/low, sinister laugh

lip curling with disgust

on an oath, his eyes popped open

purred with a predatory leer

rage boiled and rolled through (*him/her*)

said with evil satisfaction

screamed when he caught her roughly

stepped nearer closing the space between them until he could whisper harshly and be sure to be heard

sweet pleading, replaced in a blink of an eye by red-faced fury

taunted with a nasty laugh

the echo of his harsh laugh was all he left behind as he walked out of the room s

the snap of temper in (*his/her*) voice was like a lash

there was no smile in (*his/her*) voice

throttled fury filled her voice

venomous sarcasm laced every word

voice lowered to a creepy, shiver inducing whisper

wooden, distant

Additional Descriptions

a lump clogged (*his/her*) throat

angry outburst stopped (*him/her*) cold

a softer more menacing tone of voice

cleared his throat with uncharacteristic nervousness

had to swallow a couple of times before (*he/she*) could speak

heard the hunger in his own voice and forced himself to a calmer tone

hearing the desperation in (*his/her*) voice, (*he/she*) couldn't deny him

her body remembered the sound of his voice

her screams deepened, full of raw horror

her voice hooked him somewhere in the chest

(*his/her*) voice, like velvet rubbing over (*his/her*) skin

in his voice she heard a longing that echoed the burning intensity of his gaze

lost (*himself/herself*) to the compelling lilt of (*his/her*) voice

lowering his voice as he bent his head close to hers

mumbling bits and pieces of the rosary

sarcasm under that sweet smile of hers

she drew a quivering breath and started over

sound of her voice was still capable of sending rippling waves of desire through him

speaking very softly clearly not wanting the conversation to be overheard

the raspy tone was like a long, sensuous stroke down her spine

the words caught in her throat thick with an exotic accent

voice cracked over the last word

voice deepening with a powerful force

voice rough and angry with tears

wistful sound in (*his/her*) voice caught (*him/her*) off guard

words brushed along the walls of her mind like tiny butterfly wings

Laughter

Amusement, Humor

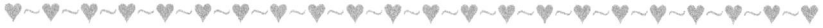

♥~♥

a little snort	bemused smile
burst out laughing	chuckle/chortle/guffaw
clearing throat	devious laugh
gasping for air	giggling
holding onto sides	huffed out a half laugh
husky laugh	hysterical laugh
jubilant shriek	making faces
loss of breath	pain in ribs or stomach
polite laugh	quirked or raised eyebrows
rough bark of laughter	shaking with laughter/hysteria
she laughed at him	slapping knee(s)
snorted a laugh	spewing food or drink
squealing	struggling to speak
tearing/wiping at eyes	trying to keep a straight face
wheezing	winking

a deep boisterous rumble that echoed through the (*forest/ room/cave*)

a full rich, very pleasant and contagious sound

a low seductive laugh escaped

a masculine mouth twitched at one end into a wry grin

by the sharp turn of her precisely shaped lips he could tell she didn't find his words amusing

caused him to choke over his coffee and slap his knee

chuckled and a deep resounding sound came from his full, sexy mouth

coughed to cover up a laugh

deep familiar chuckle strummed down her spine like caressing fingers

doubled over with laughter

faintest trace of humor lit her eyes

gave him a wink and walked off

he couldn't stop laughing long enough to get the words out

he grinned, a quick flash of undiluted charm

her gaze followed his tall broad frame up then down

her laugh was wild and touched with hysteria

his hearty laugh

his rough chuckle wickedly sensual

(*his/her*) teasing broke the tension of the moment

in his eyes she saw a glint of humor, then the amused twitch of his mouth

laughed in feminine resignation

let out a short laugh and shook (*his/her*) head

let out a squeal and giggle

pressed a hand to her chest and batted her lashes at him

roared with laughter that rumbled deep in his chest

roll(*ing, ed*) (*his/her*) eyes

shaking his head (*he/she*) chuckled as (*he/she*) slipped out of bed

sharp, and judging by his scowl, tough as nails

shot (*him/her*) a sideways look

snickered and nudged (*him/her*) with his elbow

soft laughter was a low rumble beneath her ear
the amused twitch of his mouth
uttered a soft husky laugh that charmed (*him/her*)
weak with laughter she collapsed against him

Create Your Own Tags!!!

Pain

Emotional: ache, agony, anguish, anxiety, despondency, distress, misery, shock, torment, torture, worry

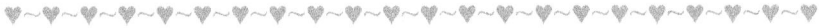

♥~♥~♥~♥~♥~♥~♥~♥~♥~♥~♥~♥~♥~♥~♥~♥~♥~♥

a dry sob burned her throat and she refused to let it out

a fragile flame of hope moved inside (*him/her*)

a heavy weight settled in (*his/her*) chest

a hot shower eased away the bruises, but couldn't wash away (*his/her*) inner turmoil

a wave of pain suffused (*his/her*) senses

been alone all (*his/her*) life, long before (*he'd/she'd*) died

calling in sick to (*work/school*)

closed (*his/her*) eyes as grief settled thick and suffocating

closed (*his/her*) eyes and tried to ignore the ache that had settled just behind (*his/her*) heart

couldn't bear to watch his warm brown eyes change from wary to horrified

didn't want to face any more memories of pain, terror and death

(*distrust/bone deep betrayal*) (*darkened/filled*) (*his/her*) gaze

face pale and haunted

felt as if (*he'd/she'd*) been gut punched and had the wind knocked out of (*him/her*)

felt the blood drain from (*his/her*) face

felt (*weary/numb/weak in the knees*)

fumbled for the zipper, hurt and anger nearly blinding her

gathered (*his/her*) defenses with several deep breaths

gave up all pretense of calm and slammed the door

gingerly fingered the photograph

had enough of the hollow grief raging inside (*him/her*)

had escaped with her virtue intact, but left her innocence behind

had no one to depend on, no one to defend (*him/her*)

(*he/she*) called in sick to (*work/school*)

(*he/she*) had an (*aching/throbbing*) pain in chest

(*he/she*) heard the rush of (*his/her*)heartbeat in ears

(*he/she*) (*rubbed/kneaded/pressed at chest*)

(*he/she*) (*wanted to be alone/avoid people*)

(*he/she*) was breaking (*his/her*) heart with the sincerity of (*his/her*) words

heart began to ache with the things (*he/she*) knew were true

heart sinking so low (*he/she*) could feel her pulse clear down to (*his/her*) toes

heart stopped, then started again with a thudding that pounded in (*his/her*) ears

hesitantly touched his fingertip to the corner of her eye, brushing away the tears

(*his/her*) appearance was unkempt

(*his/her*) heart ached for (*him/her*)

(*his/her*) (*stomach clenched/chest went tight became nauseous*)

(*his/her*) words hit (*him/her*) like body blows

(*his/her*) words stung like needles

(*his/her*) words were dagger blows straight to the jugular

huge tears rolling down her cheeks, her mouth crumpled in a wail of pain and anger

insides twisted by feelings for the woman standing before him

it was all in her beautiful, pain stricken eyes

it was (*his/her*) touch that (*he'd/she'd*) dreamed of that had kept (*him/her*) awake at night

jealousy tore through (*him/her*) like shards of glass slicing at (*his/her*) soul

keeping others at an emotional distance

kissed (*him/her*), the taste (*he'd/she'd*) longed to have again

knew the pain of (*his/her*) loss would hit (*him/her*) sooner or later

learned not to care, to never expect anything from anyone

learned young that it didn't pay to care about anyone or anything

needed someone to hold (*him/her*), kiss away (*his/her*) sorrow

old pain shimmered deep inside, blending with the fury

pain dug into (*his/her*) soul and tore at (*his/her*) last dream

pain knifed through (*him/her*), leaving (*him/her*) breathless

pain lashed at (*him/her*) stealing (*his/her*) breath

pained him to no end that he'd been the one to deliver the blow

played games with (*his/her*) emotional stability

refused to let (*him/her*) glimpse (*his/her*) vulnerability

rueful note to his final words held her rooted to the spot

screamed silently at the injustice that had brought (*him/her*) to this point in (*his/her*) life

seen his face that morning when he'd realized she had children

she froze, the smile on her face as rigid and fragile as hand-blown glass

she'd been an unwanted, unasked for responsibility

she screamed the question at him

she was going to throw up

shock dulled (*his/her*) senses

shock fused with hurt, becoming rage, turning into pain

sorrow ate at (*his/her*) soul

spirit as broken as (*his/her*) heart

(*splotchy/swollen*) face from crying

stared at (*him/her*) with wide, stunned eyes

stroked her hair and whispered soothingly until her shallow gasps evened out

swallowed an upsurge of sobs and dashed to the window

tainted by the stain of (*his/her*) illegitimate birth

taking half a step back, (*he/she*) stared at (*him/her*) in stupefied shock

taught (*himself/herself*) not to need anyone, not to depend on anyone

Texas-sized chip on his (*broad/wide/narrow*) shoulders

the air whooshed out of (*him/her*) like (*he'd/she'd*) just buried a fist in (*his/her*) stomach

the breath whooshed out of (*him/her*) as if (*he'd/she'd*) been sucker punched

the deck had been stacked against (*him/her*) since the day (*he'd/she'd*) been born

the look on (*his/her*) face couldn't have been worse if (*he'd/she'd*) driven a knife through (*his/her*) heart

the only person who'd ever loved (*him/her*) was gone

the pain was closing in on her, the weight of it crushed her

turned away and looked at the sky

vanished into the (*gray/dark*) sheet of driving rain

voice sharp as a whip, cutting into (*his/her*) skin and flaying (*his/her*) heart

words cut like a knife

worry filled (*him/her*) over (*his/her*) oath to harm or get revenge

zipped up his jeans and turned away from her

Physical: ache, agony, angry, anguish, bleeding, bloody, bruised, burn/burning, chafe, excruciating ferocious, fever, fierce, hurting, inflamed, injured, irritated, laceration, life-threatening, merciless, pulsate, piercing, raw, sensitive, severe, sharp, sore, smarting, spasm, sting/stinging, stitch, strain, suffering, tender, terrible, throb, unbearable, uncomfortable, unmerciful, vicious

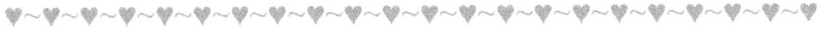

♥~♥

a fine edge of terror and pain sharpened her perceptions

a mother of a migraine

a sudden surge of weariness flooded him and he had to fight to stay on his feet

ached and hurt so much he could scarcely breathe

ached in places she'd never known she had

all he'd gotten for his efforts were bruises and broken bones

although in extreme pain, (*he/she*) was determined to stay on top of it

an explicable sorrow ate at (*his/her*) soul

awful tearing in (*his/her*) side turned a burning numbness

bit back the bile as the pain lancing through (*his/her*) head made (*him/her*) nauseous

blood and abrasions streaked (*his/her*) face, arms and legs

blood spurting from (*his/her*) (*arm/leg/shoulder*)

closed her eyes as pain tore through her

couldn't hear the words over the ringing in her ears

couldn't remember a time when (*he'd/she'd*) ached so badly

cried out at the searing burn

doubled over in pain, retching violently

eased (*his/her*) aching body into the chair

emitted a shriek and curled up on her side

every inch of his body protested as intense pain warned him not to move every muscle in (*his/her*) body cried out for relief

excruciating pain took (*his/her*) breath away

eyes filled with apology and an echo of (*his/her*) pain

felt the pressure squeezing (*his/her*) windpipe

gripped his hand as she rode the wave of pain of the contraction

had shrapnel embedded in his entire right side

her eyes cloud with pain, her hands tighten on his with a death grip

(*he/she*) felt (*cold/feverish*)

(*he/she*) felt (*faint/dizzy/like blacking out*)

(*he/she*) (*hobbled/limped/took tentative steps*)

(*he/she*) staggered and went down hard

(*he/she*) was going to walk with a limp, probably for the rest of (*his/her*) life

her teeth chattered so violently he could barely understand her

(*his/her*) expression tight with pain

(*his/her*) (*fingers shook/heart raced/blood rushed/pulsed*)

(*his/her*) muscles were (*tight/rigid*)/(*knees buckled*)

his right arm was useless, his left too weak to shoulder his weapon

(*his/her*) vision grayed

just thinking about moving sent white starbursts of pain through (*his/her*) brain

laughed bitterly as blinding pain swept through (*him/her*)

leg was badly broken

lights danced in front of (*his/her*) eyes as (*he/she*) slowly slid to the floor

lines of strain around (*his/her*) mouth had deepened

looked cold, miserable and achingly vulnerable in her nakedness muscles in (*his/her*) body ached and (*his/her*) shoulders burned with agony

nausea rolled in (*his/her*) throat and (*he/she*) bolted from the bed

pain exploded at the base of (*his/her*) skull

pain exploded through (*his/her*) limbs

pain thundered through (*his/her*) head

pain was a white hot bolt of agony

perspiring from the anticipated pain

powerful and angry, his hand grabbed her upper arm and spun her around

probed the painful area and winced

scrunched her eyes shut, grabbed her knees and pushed

(*side/leg/back/arm*) pulsing with a fiery, numbing pain

staggered and went down hard

struggled to speak, but only a groan passed (*his/her*) lips

supported (*him/her*) until the pain eased

sweat beading on (*his/her*) upper lip

the back of (*his/her*) head struck the wall

the excruciating pain in (*his/her*) middle

the pain lancing through (*his/her*) head made (*him/her*) nauseous

the stinging slap startled (*him/her*)

took a deep breath before (*he/she*) tried to lift (*his/her*) arm

tried to ignore the pain, tried not to give in to the shock and terror

tried to suck air into (*his/her*) lungs

underneath the makeshift bandage blood seeped out

unprepared for the contraction that wrapped around her belly

vision cleared to a blurred fuzziness

wondered if (*he'd/she'd*) cracked a couple of ribs
wrists were bound together, arms drawn over (*his/her*) head

Create Your Own Tags!!!

Emotions

Cheerfulness: contentment, delight, ecstasy, exhilaration, happiness, gladness, glee, joy, pleasure

Joy: bliss, buzz, contentment, delight, enjoyment, euphoria, exultation, ecstasy, elation, glee, gratification, happiness, harmony, heaven, joyfulness, jubilation, kick, merriment, paradise, pleasure, rapture, satisfaction, thrill, warmed her heart

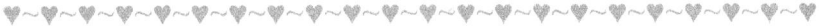

♥~♥~♥~♥~♥~♥~♥~♥~♥~♥~♥~♥~♥~♥~♥~♥~♥~♥~♥

abject gratitude at his perseverance flooded her

an hour or two of lovemaking would cure more than a couple of aches

as tears welled in his eyes, he stared down at the child he'd helped bring into the world

closed her eyes and leaned back into him

filled (*his/her*) lungs with a deep satisfying breath

(*he/she*) gave a satisfied sigh

(*he/she*) had a (*bright/optimistic outlook*)/(*glass half full*)

(*he/she*) had a light spring in (*his/her*) step

(*he/she*) had no desire to be anywhere but right here

(*he/she*) (*hummed/whistled/sang/smiled*)

(*he/she*) was at ease with (*self/world*)

he'd loved her belly when it was big with their child

he'd loved the way she'd grown heavy with his child

heart swelled at the sight of...

heavens, but the man was something to look at

her laughter bubbled over

119

her mouth trembled as she reached up to touch his face with
tentative fingers

his gait was easy and unhurried as they strolled hand in hand

(*his/her*) face, beautiful by any measure, broke into a smile

(*his/her*) mere presence brought (*him/her*) (*contentment/joy*)

(*his/her*) posture was relaxed

his praise made her feel all bubbly inside

his smile made her spirits soar with shameless delight

his warm breath fanned her face seconds before his lips
touched hers

it was a crushing homecoming as he held her

it was his rough edge and raw strength she loved best

joy burst forth in a brilliant glow of love

saw the flash of amusement behind (*his/her*) eyes

she had a tidy little inheritance from her grandfather

she had finally found a place where she was (*needed/wanted*)

she laughed at him

she sighed in delight as he swayed them back and forth

she was easily pushing her way into his heart

tears filled her eyes as light overflowed her soul

undisguised pride in her shone in his dark gaze

wiped the tears from her face, stricken with the majesty she'd
just witnessed

Confidence: buoyancy, coolness, poise, self-assured, self-reliance

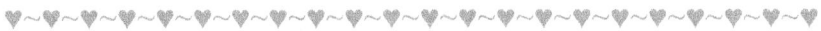

♥~♥~♥~♥~♥~♥~♥~♥~♥~♥~♥~♥~♥~♥~♥~♥~♥~♥~♥~♥

a man who could handle any situation and remain unfazed

a woman proud of both her heritage and her independence

an air of danger and intrigue about him

as long as she was with him she'd be safe

chest out, shoulders back (*he/she*) made direct eye contact

create a task force secretly operated and funded by his family's fortune

flashed her a sexy, wicked, smile both invitation and challenge

for the first time in a long time, he felt there were possibilities to be explored

from what she'd seen, he was capable of handling just about anything

gave (*him/her*) a (*knowing/playful grin/smile/wink/an easy nod*)

gave one sturdy nod that said she was ready to go

good at masking (*his/her*) real thoughts when (*he/she*) wanted to

had a pistol loaded with six silver bullets that would stop a vampire cold

he encouraged her with a slow nod

he'd played mind games plenty in his life, but this was no bluff

he'd promised to take care of her, and he would keep that promise

(*he/she*) enjoyed (*his/her*) (*light-hearted teasing/joking/telling jokes*)

he was confident his expression revealed nothing of what he was thinking

his battle instincts stirred, his senses lifting to the next level of acuity his booming laugh (*was full of confidence/drew the attention of those around them*)

his grip firm and solid, giving her the impression of controlled strength

(*his/her*) (*dainty/strong/proud*) chin lifted

laughed, slow and easy

looking people directly in the eye

made every decision with cold-blooded reason

pride elevated her chin a few notches

she knew what she wanted and wasn't shy about asking for it

she only had to reach for him with her mind

so sleek, so confident, so sure of who (*he/she*) was

taught her how to live again

the instant his arms went around her the rest of the world melted away

the lie came out smoothly

the show of authority scared the bejeebers out of her

waited with interest for his friend's reaction

walking with a swagger/sauntering

Determination: discipline, fortitude, grit, strength of mind, purpose, resolve, self-control, willpower

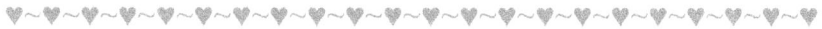

♥~♥~♥~♥~♥~♥~♥~♥~♥~♥~♥~♥~♥~♥~♥~♥~♥~♥

a mixture of tenderness and lethal determination

accepting his challenge to speak her mind

already made a mental note

another gut check and deep reach for discipline

clamped his emotions down

determined not to (*make that mistake again/turn back*)

drawing in a deep breath

emotions he'd conditioned himself not to feel

forced last night's erotic images to the back of (*his/her*) mind

gathered the broken fragments of her courage and met his gaze head on

gave (*him/her*) a pointed look

gritted his teeth together tightly, trying to keep his emotions under control

had no intention of letting (*him/her*) die for (*him/her*)

had the look of a she-wolf protecting her cub

had to know what was ticking away in that sharp brain of hers

he decided not just to have her, but to make her beg for him

her gustiness made his heart clench

(*he/she*) crossed (*his/her*) arms over (*his/her*) chest

(*he/she*) had a (*bright, positive outlook/(strong) belief in self*)

(*he/she*) (*ignored the opposition/kept focus on goal*)

(*he/she*) refused to (*give up/give in*)

(*he/she*) rubbed hands together in anticipation

his goal was to soothe and seduce her, not scare her more

his strength surrounded her, his eyes demanded she listen

hoping to quietly disappear to avoid the investigationignoring the sexual tension she felt building between them

in (*his/her*) mind (*he/she*) saw the life (*he/she*) had yet to live

jerked the steering wheel, but the tires didn't hold when (*he/she*) hit a patch of ice

keeping her safe was his obsession

liked the way concentration drew (*his/her*) heavy brows together

lived by a rigid standard of conduct

making arrangements as coldly and rationally as possible

managed to drag her hands down, forced his fingers to wrap around her wrists

planned to live the rest of his life in celibacy

reached deep for his willpower and pulled her hands gently away from him

resisted the charm in (*his/her*) voice

she was his and he wouldn't let anyone hurt her

spoke softly, trying to dispense hope and healing with (*his/her*) words

staying focused on (*his/her*) betrayal was the only way to keep (*his/her*) distance from (*him/her*)

the unblinking gaze of a hawk focused on prey

there was cop in his eyes, in his voice

thin features were tight with determination

took a cleansing breath

tried to focus on (*his/her*) face through a haze of desire

trying to look poised and relaxed

wasn't about to die for him

wasn't going to let him see a chink in her reinforced wall

wouldn't allow (*him/her*) to die if (*he/she*) could help it

Defiance: boldness, disobedience, insolence, insubordination, non-cooperation, rebelliousness

❤~❤~❤~❤~❤~❤~❤~❤~❤~❤~❤~❤~❤~❤~❤~❤~❤~❤

a jut to her jaw told him she would be a fierce enemy if crossed

angled her head to stare at his grasping hand

cut her a sharp look that dared her to argue

daring her to defy him, he invaded her personal space

defiance flashed through her eyes

defiant gleam in (*his/her*) baby-blue eyes

didn't apologize for assuming she was a brainless twit

drawing (*his/her*) back ramrod straight

felt honor-bound to hold (*his/her*) ground

(*gray/color*) eyes narrowed at the challenge in (*his/her*) voice

(*he/she*) cocked or tilted head

(*he/she*) forced a casual shrug

(*he/she*) huffed a sigh of annoyance

(*he/she*) laughed, mockery twisting (*his/her*) face

(*he/she*) (*waved hand in dismissal/walked away*)

her chin angled up and she met his gaze

he was a master at controlling conversation

(*his/her*) eyes gleamed with amused certainty

(*his/her*) (*determined walk/strut or swagger*)

(*his/her*) lips pressed thin

(*his/her*) (*raised voice/yelling/cursing/talking over people*)

his laugh was arrogant

lifted both hands in mock surrender

lifting chin/crossing arms/glowered indignantly

lips a flat line of disapproval

sat down and crossed (*his/her*) arms over his chest

standing too close/stiffening (*his/her*) shoulders

steadfastly ignoring the force of desire in his eyes

the edge in her voice stopped him

the sneer he managed not to show on his face was present in his tone of voice

the stubborn burn in her eyes infuriating him

wasn't going to let their friendship fall apart because they'd slept together

Distance: aloofness, cold, detachment, disinterest, hold back, inaccessibility, indifferent, preserve, remoteness, reserve, save, seclusion, solitude, superiority, unfriendliness

couldn't afford to care or indulge (*himself/herself*) in emotions that would only lead to disaster

drove in silence for a while, saying nothing at all

(*he/she*) (*flinched away/recoiled/avoided being touched*)

(*he/she*) refused to look at (*him/her*),(*looked down/turned away*)

his eyes narrowed and she felt him take an emotional step back

his (color) eyes were as ruthless and remote as they'd been since the day she'd betrayed him

(*his/her*) expression was (*blank/an emotionless stare*)

(*his/her*) eyes were (*cold/dead/flat*)

instead of the pain (*he/she*) sensed in (*him/her*) a moment ago, now there was just cool detachment

instinctively (*he/she*) pulled back from any kind of emotional attachment

standing in the morgue, steeling (*himself/herself*) to identify...

stared at (*him/her*) a moment, (*his/her*) expression unreadable

the fierce light in (*his/her*) eyes went out

they were God knows how many clicks behind enemy lines

was very good at being self-sufficient, at being detached

Conflict: argue, argument, be at odds, bicker, clash, collide, contradiction, controversy, disagreement, discord, discrepancy, dispute, divergence, fall-out, fight, friction, quarrel, row, spar, spat, strain, stress, tension

♥~♥

(a fake marriage/marriage of convenience) was the only thing he could think of to ensure her safety

at the use of her old nickname, she glanced *(back/up)*, startled

denial shouted through *(him/her)*, but deep inside *(he/she)* knew *(he/she)* was right

had about had it with the squeaky-clean routine

he didn't want to be gallant, he wanted to succumb to temptation

he wanted to cradle her close and tell her everything was going to be *(alright/okay)*

(his/her) mind was in turmoil, and *(his/her)* heart in an uproar

(he/she) would never be able to love the real *(him/her)*

(his/her) emotions were raw, chafed and sore

felt more than a tad of regret *(he/she)* hadn't been completely honest with *(him/her)*

it was good to be hot and bothered, but it would be nice if *(he/she)* felt the same way

looked down at her with unflinching directness

ran an agitated hand through *(his/her)* hair

senses still reeled from the experience

sucking in a shallow breath, *(he/she)* jerked *(his/her)* gaze away

the intensity of his look pounded her until she had to look away

the party-girl mask kept slipping, leaving her emotions raw, her heart (*unprotected/on display/exposed*)

tried to imagine (*himself/herself*) transforming into a wolf

what had happened between them had been entirely (*his/her*) fault

wasn't proud of the quick rush of envy

would be expected to paint on a cheerful face, to act as if everything was okay

Longing: aim, appetite, craving, desire, fancy, fondness, goal, hankering, hunger, lust, nostalgia, objective, passion, pining, target, thirst, want, yen

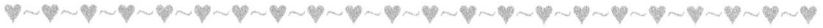

♥~♥

a completely physical, emotion-free affair was what (*he/she*) wanted

a longing unlike anything (*he'd/she'd*) ever felt or imagined

a pang of longing shot through (*him/her*)

all he'd really wanted to do was pull her into his arms and sooth her

an urge to protect her from anymore hurt washed over him

been so sure (*he'd/she'd*) be better off without (*him/her*)

forced (*himself/herself*) not to yearn for what (*he/she*) could never have

had been an eternity since he'd dared be this close to a female

(*he'd/she'd*) been fantasizing about kissing (*him/her*) for months

(*he/she*) wanted to cross the chasm that separated them

(*he/she*) wanted to pick up where they'd left off a lifetime ago

he wanted to touch her, to feel the softness of her flesh in his hand

his mouth touched hers in the darkness, her throat ached with longing just for once (*he/she*) wanted to be a normal person, have normal problems, live a normal life and love a normal (*guy/girl*)

longed to sample her full, moist lips

longed to set free her hair

(*low/soft*) voice and tender glance reminded (*him/her*) of the kiss they'd shared

missed being kissed and touched and held in a man's strong arms

more than anything (*he/she*) wanted a family of (*his/her*) own

needed him to be a good guy and love her back

never wanted anything in his life as much as he wanted to bury his face in her hair

powerful rush of emotions that made (*his/her*) throat ache with (*love/regret/need*)

she just wanted (*hero*) to be who he said he was

she missed being kissed and touched and held in a man's strong arms

swallowed hard over the sudden lump of sadness in (*his/her*) throat

there was something in (*his/her*) tone that touched a place inside (*him/her*)

wanted to cross the chasm that separated them

wanted to touch her, to feel the softness of her flesh in his hand

was hard to hope when (*his/her*) hopes had been dashed so ruthlessly in the past

watched (*him/her*) from the corner of (*his/her*) eye and felt a surge of longing and regret

when (*his/her*) arms closed around (*him/her*), it felt like (*he'd/she'd*) come home

wished (*he/she*) didn't look so damn sexy

wished (*he/she*) wouldn't tease (*him/her*) with the hope of what could possibly be

wishing he could lift some of the burden from her slender shoulders

would trade all (*his/her*) degrees for a kiss from (*him/her*)

Create Your Own Tags!!!

Surprise: admission, amaze, astonish, astound, blow, bolt from the blue, bombshell, confession, disaster, disclosure, discovery, expose, flabbergast, revelation, shock, stagger, stun, upset

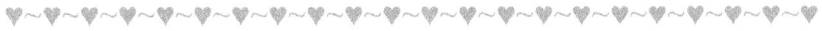

♥~♥~♥~♥~♥~♥~♥~♥~♥~♥~♥~♥~♥~♥~♥~♥~♥~♥~♥

a multitude of layers beneath the expensive veneer and buff body

a warm, protective feeling (*he/she*) didn't care to dwell on

blinked at the icy authority in his tone

blood pounded in his temples as he absorbed the stunning news

closed (*his/her*) open mouth

feminine façade hid her killer instincts

gratitude choked (*him/her*)

he appeared honest, and strangely enough interested in her

her heart beat (*increased/pounded hard*) from the unexpected surprise

her heart did a little skitter as he stepped closer

her hand flew to her chest in surprise

he stared down at her in surprise, she stared back in challenge

his hand grabbed her wrist with surprising force

(*his/her*) heart stopped, slowly (*he/she*) lifted her gaze to (*his/hers*)

(*his/her*) protective instincts staggered (*him/her*)

(*his/her*) surprise (*brought a wide smile/color to her cheeks/a quick bark of laughter/left her breathless*)

his muscles tensed under her touch

jaw dropped open in surprise

looked as thunderstruck as (*he/she*) felt

marveled at how thick and soft her hair felt against her skin

nearly tripped over his feet when he saw she wore nothing but a primly starched chef's apron she felt breathless couldn't stop her, (*gasp/squeal/scream/ yelp*) of surprise

she tore away his defenses, revealed his weaknesses

stared wide-eyed for two full seconds

stiffened in automatic defense

sucking in a shallow breath, (*he/she*) jerked (*his/her*) gaze away

sudden, blinding, intense need for (*him/her*) that overtook (*him/her*)

tears of happiness filled her eyes

the best way to stop her mouth was with his

the thing that surprised (*him/her*) was how nervous (*he/she*) was

took a lot of will power to keep her jaw from dropping

tore (*his/her*) mouth away from (*his/hers*) and stared down at (*him her*)

turned sharply at the voice behind (*him/her*)

unfamiliar tenderness swept through (*him/her*)

wanted to lean into the safety of his assurances

was completely mesmerized by the way (*his/her*) dark eyes looked straight into (*him/her*)

was still reeling from the kiss (*he'd/she'd*) laid on (*him/her*)

Aggravation: anger, annoyance, bother, difficulty, displeasure, disturbance, exasperation, frustration, hassle, impatience, infuriation, irritation, nuisance, problem, provocation, thorny problem, trouble, vexation

Frustration: aggravation, annoyance, disappointment, discontent, displeasure, dissatisfaction, disturbance, exasperation, hassle, impatience, infuriation, irritation, nuisance, pestering, provocation, stress, unhappiness

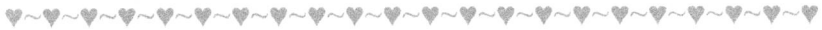

♥~♥

a muscle flicked in his jaw

after one last look at her tempting mouth, he headed out the door

a vein throbbed in his (*forehead/temple*)

behind expensive suits they were all just flesh and blood men

blew out a breath and threw (*his/her*) hands wide

didn't have too many exploitable weaknesses

exasperation and a sense of hopeless futility pounded through (*him/her*)

expression plainly said as far as (*he/she*) was concerned, (*he/she*) could go to hell

face bone white with fury and frustration

folded his tanned muscular arms across his chest

frustration and curiosity did a dangerous dance inside (*him/her*)

gave a mock sigh of relief

glanced at (*his/her*) watch and (*frowned/grimaced/scowled*)

(*he/she*) (*flicked gaze upward/cocked head/grimaced/sneered/ frowned/ground teeth together/clenched jaw/tapped foot*)

(*he/she*) gushed like every other fan (*he'd/she'd*) met

(*he/she*) let out (*a sigh/an exaggerated/frustrated sigh*)

(*he/she*) threw hands up in frustration

(*he'd/she'd*) already looked deep in (*his/her*) eyes and done something foolish once

(*his/her*) expression was pinched

(*his/her*) (*eyebrows rose/eyes narrowed/gave a blank stare*)

it wasn't his arrogance that got to her, but her reaction to him

right now what (*he/she*) wanted most was a chance to kiss (*him/her*)

scrubbed a hand across (*his face/at the roughened stubble on his chin*) in frustration

shrugged (*his/her*) shoulders in an infuriating mockery of disinterest

shrugged (*his/her*) thin shoulders

sighed and leaned forward

strong arms tugged her close

the heat from his grip and the impact of his smile seeped into her blood

took a deep breath, braced (*himself/herself*) and turned around

was annoyed but hid it with a careless shrug

weakened (*his/her*) resolve with a (*look/kiss/smile*)

when (*he/she*) saw (*person*) strolling toward (*him/her*) in the pale, early morning light, (*he/she*) swore softly

wished she could quench her craving for his body and then drop him cold

wishing he could take her into his arms and hold her

Fatigue: apathy, collapse, disillusionment, drowsiness, exhaustion, lethargy, sleepiness, sluggishness, stupor, tiredness, weakness, weariness

♥~♥

adrenaline left (*his/her*) body in a rush

all (*he/she*) wanted was peace

allowed (*himself/herself*) a moment or two of reverent reflection

braced (*his/her*) hands against the shower wall and let the warm water flow over (*him/her*)

caught her as she staggered

dark smudges of exhaustion lay under (*his/her*) eyes

dizziness swept over (*him/her*) and (*he/she*) swayed, a hand going to (*his/her*) head

drowsy thoughts focused on the conversation

every bone and muscle throbbed with tension

exhaustion taking over, pushing out all her worries and fears

expelled a long, tired breath

(*he/she*) had (*bags or circles under eyes/lack of appetite*)

(*he/she*) had (*scratchy/gritty eyes/blurred vision/heavy lids/ bloodshot/red-rimmed eyes/vacant stare/inability to focus*)

(*he she*) had (*slowed reaction time/slowed speech/heaviness in limbs/forgetfulness/impaired judgment*)

(*he/she*) pinched the bridge of (*his/her*) nose/rubbed at (*his/her*)face

(*he/she*) was barely able to keep (*his/her*) eyes open

(*he/she*) was so exhausted (*he/she*) could barely focus on the meal in front of (*him/her*)

(*he/she)* yawned involuntarily

(*his/her*) eyes drifted shut

(*his/her*) strength flowed away like water down a drain

his wrinkled unkempt, unshaved appearance filled her with worry

lines around (*his/her*) mouth, deep and drawn

muscles trembled like a newborn baby

(*numbers/details*) flew through her mind as she drifted off to sleep

slid (*his/her*) reading glasses off (*his/her*) nose and rubbed (*his/her*) temples

swayed as (*he/she*) stood

sweat broke out on (*his/her*) brow

the stitch in (*his/her*) side forced (*him/her*) to slow down

tone became gentler, resigned, as though beaten down by sudden fatigue

was good for her to rest; she'd been through so much

wasted so many nights crying into her pillow over him

Exasperation: anger, annoyance, bother, frustration, impatience, irritant, irritation, nuisance, pain, pest
♥~♥~♥~♥~♥~♥~♥~♥~♥~♥~♥~♥~♥~♥~♥~♥~♥~♥~♥

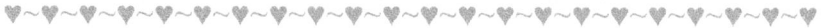

clenched his jaw as he struggled to contain the argument simmering between them

closing (*his/her*) eyes (*he/she*) drew in a slow calming breath

crossing (*his/her*) arms (*across/over*) (*his/her*) chest

damn him for being so big, making her feel so tiny and helpless

dating, bonding and making love weren't going to be enough

firmly shut her mouth

forcing (*himself/herself*) to calm down

frustration spilled out in a fiery sigh

(*he/she*) gave an exaggerated sigh

(*he/she*) held (*his/her*) head in (*his/her*) hands

(*he/she*) tapped (*his/her*) foot

(*he/she*) threw hands up

(*his/her*) attitude and actions seemed designed to perpetuate the assumption they were an item

(*his/her*) expression was pinched

(*his/her*) lips were (*blade thin/pinched tight*)

his mere presence made her feel small, insignificant and defenseless

(*his/her*) response was curt, delivered in a cool distant tone

judging by his arrogant stance, he was too cocksure of his appeal

let loose a breath that was half frustration, half disbelief

made a growling sound in his throat

met (*his/her*) question with one of (*his/her*) own

people seeing them together would think they were an item

rubbed (*his/her*) hand over (*his/her*) face

rubbing brow to ward off a headache

shoved his hat back and rubbed a hand across his eyes

stared at (*him/her*) like (*he/she*) was a fresh piece of meat

swore silently at (*him/her*) for disturbing a mental musing

the amusement (*he/she*) saw in (*his/her*) eyes made (*him/her*) stiffen

with a heavy sigh, he sat back

with a sigh (*he/she*) took another long sip of (*his/her*) drink

Confusion: bewilderment, chaos, commotion, disorder, mayhem, misunderstanding, muddle, mystification, perplexity, puzzlement, turmoil, uncertainty, upheaval, worry

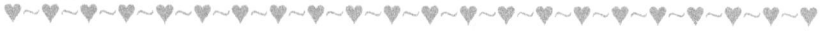

♥~♥~♥~♥~♥~♥~♥~♥~♥~♥~♥~♥~♥~♥~♥~♥~♥~♥~♥

all her questions and confusion were wiped away when his mouth closed over hers

awoke confused, with a splitting headache

chewed worriedly on her lower lip

confused (*he/she*) shook her head over (*his/her*) (*slack expression /blank look*)

could see the battle going on inside (*him/her*)

felt off-center with the world

frowning, (*he/she*) tried to find the words to explain how (*he/she*) felt

had no clear vision of where (*he/she*) wanted their relationship to go

(*he/she*) had to repeat the question

her eyes widened, sparkling with shock and something else

(*his/her*) lack of control was so out of character

(*his/her*) (*mind churned/worked rapidly*)

(*his/her*) response to the question was delayed

(*his/her*) suspicions hurt and left (*him/her*) feeling betrayed

met (*his/her*) steady gaze, then quickly glanced away

mouth felt full of cotton and (*he/she*) was painfully thirsty

response was curt, delivered in a cool distant tone

the fog had begun to lift from (*his/her*) brain

their relationship was over and (*he/she*) didn't know why

turned her face to the window glad the darkness would hide her emotions

whipped around to face (*him/her*)

wondered at the reasons that made her run like a child into his arms

wreaked havoc on (*his/her*) (*body/soul*) that (*he/she*) couldn't (*explain/understand*)

Anxiety: apprehension, concern, disquiet, fear, fretfulness, nervousness, tension, unease, worry

Fear: alarm, anxiety, apprehension, be afraid, be alarmed, be anxious, concern, dread, fright, frightened, horror, nightmare, panic, phobia, scared, tension, terrified, terror, trepidation, worry

Tension: anxiety, apprehension, fear, nervousness, pressure, strain, stress, worry

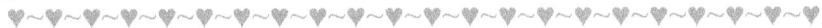

❤~❤~❤~❤~❤~❤~❤~❤~❤~❤~❤~❤~❤~❤~❤~❤~❤~❤~❤~❤

afraid he'd be put in a cage from which he would never escape

after a desperate day of fear and worry

alarm came into her eyes darkening that lovely (*gray/brown*)

angry snarl curled his lips

bit off the urge to scream

blinked rapidly as blinding light sent (*him/her*) to (*his/her*) knees

brittle, jagged pieces of the nightmare slid through (*his/her*) brain

chin quivered as she swallowed hard

could feel (*his/her*) power rise in a silent battle of wills

could feel the animosity that hummed between them

could feel time dwindling

felt slow, clumsy and stiff

felt the blood drain from her face

fought the nausea that climbed up (*his/her*) throat

fought the urge to turn and bolt

fought to even her breathing

gnawed on a ragged thumbnail

goose flesh rippling up her back

gun held level to (*his/her*) chest

had no idea why (*he/she*) suddenly couldn't breathe

hairs on the backs of (*his/her*) arms rose

heard the edge of hysteria in her voice

heart froze as (*he/she*) saw the bloody handprint on the door casing

heart pounding, knees shaking

heart pounding painfully hard

he grinned with a malevolence that turned her blood to ice water

her (*face went dead white/her blood turned to ice/her hands were frozen*)

her (*skin crawled/hackles rose*)

(*he/she*) (*cringed/flinched/gasped/recoiled/tensed up/jerked awake*)

his body wire tight as a bow string

his face bore the wrath of hell as he pushed past her

(*his/her*) gut clenched with one of (*his/her*) intuitions that never presaged anything good

(*his/her*) voice shook

just a few more steps and she'd reach the door

loomed over her tall, dark and deadly

nerves dancing in her stomach

nerves made (*his/her*) hands unsteady

nervous sweat slicked (*his/her*) body

never seen a more chilling smile

nothing but the sound of (*his/her*) breathing, quick and shallow pain sharp and jabbing, like an icicle lodged in (*his/her*) stomach

praying (*he/she*) wouldn't see how badly (*his/her*) hands were shaking

pressed a hand to her mouth

rush of (*regret/wrenching fear*)

sank to her knees, sick and shaken

sat against the wall with her eyes shut and knees drawn up to her chest

scrambled back until her shoulders hit the wall

scream tore through the air

screamed and kept screaming until her voice broke

she'd moved from location to location, but somehow he always found her

she (*edged away from him/huddled against the wall/ shuddered/trembled*)

shot from full sleep to wakefulness

sick fear coiled in the pit of (*his/her*) stomach

skin crawled as (*he/she*) looked into the big man's face

sound lodged in her throat along with her heart

stood in the shadows, trembling, then threw on the light

sweat popped out on his face and ran cold and fast from his armpits

tearing flesh as (*he/she*) struggled against the bonds

terror was a new sensation to (*him/her*)

the calm in his eyes more frightening than if he'd shouted at her

the rest of her words died in (*his/her*) throat as (*he/she*) found (*himself/herself*) face-to-face with...

there was horror in her eyes as she stared down

the violence in his eyes had her taking a step back

thoughts leaped feverously

took a deep breath against the panic
unable to evade, she went still as a cornered animal
voice shook and she made herself slow down

Create Your Own Tags!!!

Caution: alarm, alertness, apprehension, care, carefulness, caution, concern, diffidence, discretion, disquiet, distress, fear, good sense, heed, lack of confidence, mind, prudence, suspicion, think about, trepidation, unease, vigilance, wariness, watchfulness, worry

Insecurity: anxiety, apprehension, apprehensiveness, coyness, doubt, fear, fretfulness, hesitancy, indecision, insecurity, nervousness, quietness, reserve, shyness, timidity, uncertainty, unease

Uneasiness: agitation, agonize, alarm, anxiety, apprehension, awkwardness, be anxious, be concerned, clumsiness, concern, discomfort, disquiet, fear, foreboding, fret, gracelessness, hesitation, impatience, ineptness, nervousness, restlessness, unease, unrest, worry

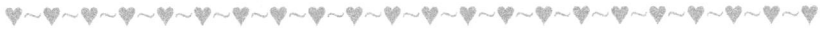

♥~♥~♥~♥~♥~♥~♥~♥~♥~♥~♥~♥~♥~♥~♥~♥~♥~♥

a ping of caution erupted in (*his/her*) chest

a whisper of unease teased (*his/her*) senses

a sensation of tender concern slipped into his mind

admitting her desire with the hope it wasn't one-sided eased the worry in her chest

being worried caused her to (*chew on fingernail/bite lip/have panic attacks/be unnaturally quiet*)

braced himself against the lure of her brazenness and her bold request

careful not to disturb the scene, (*he/she*) crouched beside the body

cautiously (*he/she*) circled it, studying it from all sides

closed like a fist around (*his/her*) heart

desperation gave (*him/her*) strength

every nerve in (*his/her*) body shrieked to get to (*him/her*)

expression filled with uneasy worry

eyes flickered warily

gauged (*his/her*) reaction carefully

gently pried (*his/her*) fingers open

he prowled, his muscled frame moving soundlessly

her nervousness touched him bone deep

(*he/she*) pushed (*his/her*) food around on the plate

hesitated for a moment, seemed to choose (*his/her*) words carefully

(*his/her*) scrutiny made (*him/her*) uncomfortable

hit with a nauseating wave

ignored the quick twist in (*his/her*) gut

it gave (*him/her*) a chill to study it

keen sense of awareness kept (*him/her*) edgy and alert

kept (*his/her*) voice chilly, (*his/her*) expression distant

let (*his/her*) gaze rake the room

narrowed (*his/her*) assessing gaze even more

she couldn't seem to stop the (*nervous laughter/illogical fears/ shifting in chair*)

silence as thick as mud oozed between them

something about (*his/her*) behavior struck (*him/her*) as odd

spoke with a quiet certainty in his voice that stopped her cold

still couldn't sleep with the lights off

stopped at the edge of the frigid river uncertain how strong the current was

the first trace of nervousness flitted across her face

the frantic holding onto a sliver of hope

the idea weaved an unsettling path through (*his/her*) consciousness

though it cost (*him/her*) some to admit the truth, (*he/she*) gave it to (*him/her*) anyway

tried to see past the image of (*his/her*) own face reflected in the mirrored lenses

uncertainty made her voice shake

wanted to forget what (*he'd/she'd*) seen

wanted to turn and walk out

was restless and needed a sense of normalcy

wiped (*his/her*) damp palms on the thighs of (*his/her*) jeans

worry wrinkled (*his/her*) brow

Guilt: blame, burden, fault, liability, responsibility, shame, troubled

Regret: apologetic, atonement, be sorry, distress, remorse, repentance, sadness, shame, sorrow

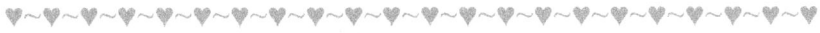

❤~❤~❤~❤~❤~❤~❤~❤~❤~❤~❤~❤~❤~❤~❤~❤~❤~❤~❤~❤

abruptly (*hero/heroine*) changed the subject

all (*he/she*) would have had to do was cut (*him/her*) loose

a pang of remorse shot through (*him/her*)

a shake of (*his/her*) head, and a long exhale

as much as (*he'd/she'd*) like to play along with the fantasy, (*he/she*) wouldn't

bit back the sob rattling in her chest

(*blue/velvet*) eyes gazed into hers with all the hypnotic intensity she remembered

closed (*his/her*) eyes, it hurt too much to look at (*him/her*)

could have spared (*him/her*) all those long weeks of suffering

could think of a hundred things that might go wrong

couldn't bring (*himself/herself*) to turn away from (*him/her*) again

couldn't face (*him/her*) anymore

done such a good job of breaking her heart and wrecking her life he could never go back

everything she'd fantasized about in a man, (*intelligent/kind/strong*)

felt a need to make up to (*him/her*) for what (*he'd/she'd*) done to (*him/her*)

felt (*his/her*) (*cheeks/ears/neck*) (*heat/burn/flame*)

for (*ten/however many*) years (*he'd/she'd*) wrestled with what happened that night

guilt rolled through (*him/her*) like hot lava

he couldn't keep her forever and he knew it

(*he/she*) felt (*his/her*) self retreating inward

(*he/she*) gave a half-hearted shrug

(*he/she*) looked (*down or away*), unable to make eye contact

(*he/she*) ought to apologize for hurting (*him/her*) so badly

he'd been a complete schmuck without even realizing it

his need to keep her safe overrode every reasonable thought

horror and guilt rose inside (*him/her*) flaying (*his/her*) soul

if only he were real, she could fall for him like a ton of bricks

if only (*he'd/she'd*) known (*him/her*) before (*he'd/she'd*) had to make that decision

if only she could erase some of her mistakes

instinct took over at one glimpse of the face that had haunted (*him/her*) for the past (*twelve/however many*) years

it wasn't as if (*his/her*) opinion of him could go any lower

last night was a huge mistake (*he/she*) couldn't let happen again

memory washed over (*him/her*) of their unforgettable night together

no way could (*he/she*) face the only (*man/woman*) (*he'd/she'd*) ever loved old feelings and memories flooded (*him/her*), catching (*him/her*) off guard

rather have the (*man/woman*) (*he/she*) loved alive and hating (*his/her*) guts than dead

released her and staggered back a step

she looked up at the man she'd loved and hated enough to die for

she wanted him; it was a miracle—and he wasn't going to turn away from it or her

she'd tried everything to get over him, but nothing had worked

should tell (*him/her*) now before their relationship went any further

sick guilt rolled through (*him/her*) like hot lava

the memory of it overpowered (*him/her*) every time (*he/she*) stepped into...

thought (*he'd/she'd*) done a noble thing to suck up (*his/her*) pain and leave (*him/her*) alone

was closer to the truth than (*he/she*) knew

was it guilt (*he/she*) felt or real affection for (*him/her*)

wasn't every day a (*guy/girl*) had to miss (*his/her*) best friend's wedding on account of a (*man/woman*)

would get them out of there and then he'd get on with his life

years of secrets, of hiding the truth weighed on (*his/her*) shoulders with back breaking force

Anger: annoyance, antagonism, fury, irritation, rage, resentment

Rage: anger, blow your top, boil with rage, frenzy, fume, fury, ire, rant and rave, seethe, storm, temper, thunder, wrath

♥~♥~♥~♥~♥~♥~♥~♥~♥~♥~♥~♥~♥~♥~♥~♥~♥~♥~♥

a black rage that bubbled in the blood

a crimson haze surrounded (*his/her*) vision

a flare of anger lanced through (*his/her*) lust

a muscle jumped in his jaw

a neatly buried, deep-down, fury settled at the corners of (*his/her*) heart

a shimmering wave of pulsing fury clouded everything

a small vein throbbed over one eyebrow

a vein near his left eye bulged as his face grew red

a vein pulsed at the base of his throat

anger narrowed his eyes, stiffened his jaw

anger poured through (*him/her*), boiling (*his/her*) blood and clouding (*his/her*) brain

anger splintered and flashed like a warning beacon

argued hotly in (*his/her*) own defense

attacked his food with short quick movements that were almost vicious

beneath the calm lay an edge of fury and frustration

(*chocolate brown/hazel/blue*) eyes bored into her

climbed to his feet, driven by an unrelenting fury

confused by (*his/her*) admission

couldn't keep the venom from (*his/her*) voice

couldn't stop the raw fury that knotted (*his/her*) gut every time (*he/she*) thought about it

curl of anger in (*his/her*) gut

cursed softly between (*his/her*) breath

dark and hot, eyes narrowed, (*his/her*) gaze locked on (*his/her*) face

deep, rough, edged with deadly calm

drilled an index finger into his chest

easily dodged her swiftly raised knee

every harsh question made (*him/her*) flinch

evil intentions distorted (*his/her*) usually reserved face

eyes narrowed and not quite sane

face turned a deep scarlet

felt (*his/her*) temper rise, but worked to keep it in check

felt the old fury rise up inside

felt the violence radiating off of him

fist slammed the desk with rage

fury came over him in a wave

fury pounded and rippled in time to the beating of (*his/her*) heart

gripping the cup more tightly, (*he/she*) tore (*his/her*) gaze away

gritted his teeth and fought down the snarl of anger nearly choking him

held up a hand in restraint, as if warning (*him/her*) off

her hand cracked against his cheek before she could stop it

(*he/she*) (*mentally counted to ten/wanted to shake*) (*him/her*)

(*he/she*) (*scowled/sneered/frowned/yelled/snapped at people*)

(*he/she*) slammed the door shut

(*he/she*) was stunned by (*his/her*) her rage

her words were whispered, but laced with vehemence

his back teeth ground together

his face reddened, a low hum of furry escaped

(*his/her*) body hummed with a fury that had (*him/her*) trembling

(*his/her*) doubting expression was really beginning to piss (*him/her*) off

(*his/her*) fuse was short and burning

(*his/her*) hand tightened on phone

(*his/her*) (*hands balled into fists/fisted in*) (*his/her*) pockets

(*his/her*) nostrils flared

his hard corded body vibrated with tension

his fists clenched at his sides

his whole body tightening as though a statue of fear and anger

hit the door with the flat of his hand

ignored the voice of caution growing louder by the heart beat

insult flashed across (*his/her*) face

impatience fired a spark of temper in (*his/her*) eyes

in one smooth, angry motion, (*he/she*) rose and moved to the door

knowing (*he/she*) needed a clear head, (*he/she*) fought back the anger

letting the fury roll off (*him/her*)

lips drawn back in a silent snarl

mouth was pressed into a tight line

moved into an openly protective stance

narrowed (*hard/cold/flinty*) eyes on (*him/her*)

paced around (*him/her*) in a tight circle

(*pound/slam*) fist into (*door/cupboard/wall*)

punching/kicking/throwing things

rage shined in (*his/her*) eyes

stared down at her with smoldering intensity

sudden urge to pitch the phone across the room

taut line of his jaw, the feral expression in his eyes

the faint tinge of black and blue next to one of her eyes was like a sucker punch to the gut

the one sign he'd shown of temper was that jaw twitch

the pistol shook in (*his/her*) hand as (*he/she*) tried to take aim

there was nothing inside but an endless burning thirst for revenge

the situation demanded immediate (*action/attention*)

the sudden tensing of her fine jaw

the thought sent a thrill of pure rage through (*him/her*)

the warning tone of his voice deep and angry

their gazes battled for long moments

took her shoulders in his hands

tuck the anger back inside and follow orders

turned on (*him/her*), (*his/her*) eyes flashing

turning (*his/her*) back on (*him/her*) in fury

violent images lurched obscenely inside (*his/her*) skull

voice was low and trembling with anger

voice was sharp and low

Disgrace: degradation, dishonor, embarrassment, humiliation, mortification, shame

Embarrassment: awkwardness, chagrin, degradation, discomfiture, disgrace, dishonor, humiliation, loss of face, mortification, shame, unease

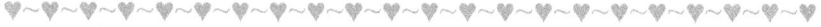

♥~♥~♥~♥~♥~♥~♥~♥~♥~♥~♥~♥~♥~♥~♥~♥~♥~♥~♥~♥

a hot wave of shame, unexpected, unwanted, washed over (*him/her*)

ashamed that (*he/she*) knew how badly (*he/she*) wanted (*him/her*)

brutal hands cruising over her body

could feel (*his/her*) heart throbbing in (*his/her*) flushed cheeks

could hardly force (*himself/herself*) to meet (*his/her*) gaze

didn't like the feeling (*he'd/she'd*) been played

doubted (*he/she*) could look (*him/her*) in the face without showing guilt

embarrassment flooded through her when the desk clerk asked what type of room they wanted

felt (*his/her*) cheeks burn

felt the burn of (*his/her*) gaze as it fixed on (*his/hers*)

filled with embarrassed discomfort

fought the urge to squirm under (*his/her*) mother-in-law's narrow-eyed stare

hating the instant memory of him kissing her so provocatively

(*he/she*) (*blamed another/deflected attention away from self*)

(*he/she*) (*cleared throat/pretended to not hear/see*)

(*he/she*) ducked (*his/her*) head

(*he/she*) (*fidgeted/rubbed neck/squirmed*)

(*he/she*) (*stammered/stuttered/was speechlessness*)

(*he'd/she'd*) never been in a situation like this before

hid (*his/her*) face

(*his/her*) chest heaved as (*he/she*) began to weep

(*his/her*) face was heating in a blush, as if (*he/she*) were fourteen

(*his/her*) gaze clashed with (*his/hers*), startled and upset

holding her head up high despite the look of pure disdain from the women

it was the first time another man other than her husband had touched her

knew (*he'd/she'd*) seen something in (*his/her*) eyes that embarrassed (*him/her*)

mortified at unconsciously seeking his heat and shelter while she slept

sat up slowly and reached for (*his/her*) head to keep the room from spinning

sent (*him/her*) a startled glance before falling silent

stared at (*him/her*) silently for a minute, then cleared (*his/her*) throat

the thought of being only one in a long succession of women he'd enjoyed, stabbed at her

Anguish: agony, angst, despair, distress, grief, pain, sorrow, suffering, torment, torture

Defeat: annihilate, beat, confound, conquer, cream, crush, despair, flay, flog, get the better of, lash, overawe, overcome, overpower, overshadow, overwhelm, rout, slaughter, spank, squash, subdue, surmount, surrender, thrash, triumph over, trounce, vanquish, whitewash, whip

Despair: anguish, defeat, dejection, depression, desolation, desperation, despondency, gloom, hopelessness, lose heart, lose hope, misery

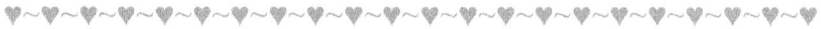

♥~♥~♥~♥~♥~♥~♥~♥~♥~♥~♥~♥~♥~♥~♥~♥~♥~♥

a pit of hopelessness opened in (*his/her*) stomach

chin trembled ever so slightly

clenched (*his/her*) teeth against the wave of hopeless, bitter pain

desperation gave (*him/her*) strength

face etched with sorrow

felt tears prick her eyes at the thought of seeing him

felt the twist deep in (*his/her*) heart

fought down the urge to comfort (*him/her*)

hated the despair she saw in her own eyes

he regretted (*his/her*) cruelty instantly

her voice was nothing more than a broken whisper

(*he/she*) was at a loss for words

(*he/she*) whispered, (*his/her*) voice miserable

he'd grown up hard and tough and just a little mean

(*he/she*) knew there was no changing the past

(*he'd/she'd*) lost people in (*his/her*) life

her eyes (*closed/squeezed/shut*)

it hurt to see (*his/her*) pained expression

it made him hurt to see (*his/her*) face so ravaged by emotion

154

it was time to stop looking back and clinging to those memories

knees buckled and (*he/she*) sank into the nearest chair

no more than a blip in (*his/her*) memories

now (*he/she*) could only contemplate what might have been

out of money and not a soul on earth to call for help

pulled herself into a miserable ball of shame

reaching out to steady self

she stumbled mid-stride

she was (*crying/sobbing/wailing*)

she was (*inconsolable/unable to eat/sleep*)

stood with (*his/her*) head down, a (*man/woman*) emotionally exhausted

struggled to keep the desperation out of (*his/her*) voice

the bitter agony that welled inside (*him/her*) was crippling

words slipped out painfully from between tightly clenched teeth

Disappointment: displeasure, dissatisfaction, discontent, disillusionment, disapproval, bitterness, world-weariness, regret

Disillusionment: bitterness, disappointment, disapproval, discontent, disillusionment, displeasure, dissatisfaction, regret, rejection, world-weariness

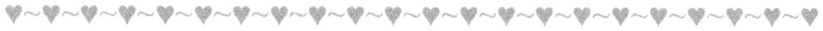

♥~♥~♥~♥~♥~♥~♥~♥~♥~♥~♥~♥~♥~♥~♥~♥~♥~♥~♥

all (*his/her*) life (*he'd/she'd*) never felt (*he'd/she'd*) measured up to her father's expectations/to (*his/her*) potential

an aching heart and empty arms

believed in honesty and integrity, but over the last few years had developed serious trust issues

blew out a breath and backed another step away from (*him/her*)

constant disappointment to the (*family/father/mother*) (*he'd/she'd*) wanted to please most

could feel the rejection coming off (*him/her*) in waves

couldn't disguise the doubt in (*his/her*) eyes

didn't have time for a relationship

disappointed (*he'd/she'd*) made no move to capture their earlier closeness

forced (*himself/herself*) not to yearn for what (*he/she*) could never have

(*he/she*) blew out a breath and backed another step away from (*him/her*)

(*he'd/she'd*) once believed in honesty and integrity

(*he/she*) (*hesitated/paced*)

(*he/she*) made a big show of looking disappointed

(*he/she*) reached up and unhooked (*his/her*) arms from around (*his/her*) neck

(*he/she*) rubbed at (*forehead/temples*)

(*his/her*) (*false cheer/weak smile*)

(*his/her*) heart sank

(*his/her*) shoulders (*slumped/sagged/drooped*)

incredible surging joy, (*he'd/she'd*) always thought this moment would bring didn't come

it was the first time (*he'd/she'd*) allowed (*himself/herself*) to form the thought, but once it was there (*he/she*) knew it to be true

over the last few years (*he'd/she'd*) developed serious trust issues

reaching(*ed*) out to steady (*his/her*) *self*

she'd sworn off smooth talking, shallow playboys who had no more muscle than brain

she hated the assumptions that came with her looks

so many chances to connect had already passed them by

the ball of need in her gut iced over in reaction to his obvious ego

the change of expression was a cooling, a withdrawal

their meeting had been less than friendly

unmistakable regret in (*his/her*) tone

was disappointed (*he'd/she'd*) made no move to capture their earlier closeness

was the first time (*he'd/she'd*) allowed (*himself/herself*) to remember their past

Unhappiness

♥~♥

agony	dejection	depression
desolation	despair	despondent
discontent	gloom	grief
melancholy	misfortune	misery
sadness	sorrow	tears/woe
wretchedness		

Tears

♥~♥

bawl	blubber	cry
howl	moan	shed tears
snivel	snuffle	sob
wail	weep	whimper

blue eyes wide with shock, lips trembling

closed her eyes, willing herself not to cry

cried herself to sleep

distinct sadness in (*his/her*) eyes

eyes bloodshot from hours of crying

eyes moist with joy

eyes red-rimmed and swimming with constant tears

hard wrenching sobs filled the room

(*he/she*) swallowed hard, nodded, not trusting (*his/her*) voice

(*he/she*) swiped at the tears with the balls of (*his/her*) thumbs

her vision wavered behind unshed tears

her whimpers escalated into loud heaving sobs

(*his/her*) eyes clouded and (*he/she*) looked away

(*his/her*) tears slipped free and (*he/she*) dropped (*his/her*) head into (*his/her*) hands

kissed the salty tears from her cheeks

paced the room, wringing her hands as tears streamed

realized she was fighting tears

sobs reduced to sniffles and tears

tears burned her cheeks with their heat and quiet power

tears burned the back of (*his/her*) throat

tears flowed hot and humiliating

tears of frustration that he wasn't being forthcoming with her coursed down her face

tears left clean tracks in the soot on her face

thin bitter tears of terror

unshed tears blurred (*his/her*) vision

Additional Emotions

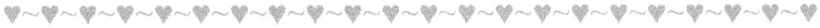

after a brief mental tussle between his half angel, half devil conscience

a tiny spark whispered in (*his/her*) brain (*he/she*) was being irrational

distracted from (*his/her*) memories by the warmth in (*his/her*) voice

drew a bolstering breath

flirting playfully, harmlessly

frowning, (*he/she*) tried to find the words to explain how (*he/she*) felt

(*he'd/she'd*) been flirting playfully, harmlessly

(*he/she*) didn't offer any false promises

hope hit (*him/her*) in the chest, taking (*his/her*) breath away

never seen anyone as completely in-your-face honest

swallowed past the knot of emotion lodged in (*his/her*) throat

swallowing a knot of something unexpected wedged in (*his/her*) throat

the sickening feeling of free fall just under (*his/her*) stomach

the twist of jealousy was ridiculous

the woman in front of him brought out his primitive instinct to protect

took the note of disbelief as a compliment

wished for a fleeting moment, that (*he/she*) was half the (*man/woman*) (*he/she*) seemed to think (*he/she*) was

was the kind of (*man/woman*) who dealt in revenge

Create Your Own Tags!!!

Bonus Extras

Acceptance

♥~♥

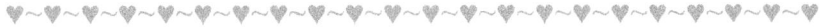

any relationship (*he/she*) had with (*him/her*) could only be casual

bitter experience told (*him/her*) (*he/she*) would get over (*his/her*) infatuation with (*him/her*) soon enough

didn't have too many exploitable weaknesses

didn't trust (*his/her*) own reaction to (*his/her*) closeness

didn't trust (*himself/herself*) to react

felt even more foolish when he saw the light of understanding in her big, dark eyes

for several surprised seconds (*he/she*) stared at (*him/her*)

given a task (*he/she*) would do a good job; given an order (*he/she*) would rebel

good at extracting revenge, it was one of (*his/her*) secret pleasures

had displayed an understanding and sensitivity for which (*he/she*) was extremely grateful

hadn't said a sincere prayer since (*he/she*) was (*eight/whatever age*)-years old

he could walk, talk, even kill in utter silence

he didn't lie well, half truths and evasion suited him better

he didn't want him to carry her again

(*he/she*) was disturbing both mentally and physically

(*he/she*) wasn't the same (*man/woman*) (*he/she*) was when (*he'd/she'd*) started this adventure

161

(*he'd/she'd*) been written off as a (*man/woman*) without a future, because (*he/she*) was a (*man/woman*) who had no past

he'd kissed her and the hole he'd been digging for himself went a lot deeper

his hand was capable of killing, yet it touched her gently

if they were connected, she would know the moment he opened his eyes

knew in a split second why so many girls in town found him dangerously sexy

knew pushing her too hard, too fast would be a huge mistake on his part, so he held back

lay tensely waiting for (*him/her*) to make the next move

like looking at a mirror image of what (*he/she*) felt

made the mistake of meeting (*his/her*) eyes and the burn of heat in their shadowed depths

measured himself by skills mastered or missions accomplished

no more fantasies about (*him/her*) because somehow or other (*he'd/she'd*) become too important to (*him/her*) already

one look into the intruder's eyes and (*he/she*) changed (*his/her*) mind

remind herself how far (*he'd/she'd*) come from the poor little orphan to the (*man/woman*) (*he/she*) was today

she didn't try to touch him, his stance was too rigid for that

she'd humiliated him and that couldn't go unpunished

that intense sexual attraction had nothing to do with long-term capability

the pendant would protect her

this (*man/woman*) could hurt (*him/her*) in a way like no other

touching her like that screamed of impropriety

understanding beckoned, like a glimmer of light beneath a lifting fog

would take advantage of every doubt, every weakness

Curiosity, Intrigue

♥~♥

didn't know what had come over (*him/her*), but whatever it was, (*he/she*) aimed to take full advantage of it

(*he/she*) was bluffing—(*he/she*) felt it around the edges of (*his/her*) consciousness

(*his/her*) body, (*his/her*) entire being was acutely aware

(*his/her*) expression carefully neutral, (*he/she*) kept his gaze on hers and waited

his scent, his aura and his tough masculine persona hooked her

in sleep she had a childlike vulnerability

made (*himself/herself*) completely unreadable

never been the kind of man to deny himself carnal pleasures

perplexed by the sharp stab of jealousy

she'd captivated the attention of every male around

was a woman who made no effort at all to be sexy

was an unspoken secret around town why (*he'd/she'd*) left

wasn't the kind of (*man/woman*) who normally drew (*his/her*) interest

wondered what kind of future they would have together

Thoughts

♥~♥

a brief fling would be too intense, fierce, hot, consuming

all she could think about was raking her fingers through his (*color*) hair and rubbing her body up against his

be lying to (*himself/herself*) if (*he/she*) denied there was chemistry between them

been too busy over the last couple of years to even fantasize about sex

considered (*himself/herself*) a sensible (*man/woman*)

163

could see where this was heading...straight down a (*path/road*) that ended with (*him/her*) getting (*screwed/worked*) over

determined not to give way to her fears, she met his eyes

dreamed of coming home to a comfy house, a loving (*husband/ wife*) and the sound of children

filled with self-doubt and bitterness

fortunately (*he/she*) could work dancing as a form of seduction

had been a long time since (*he'd/she'd*) been with a (*man/ woman*)

had no choice but to forget (*him/her*)

(*he/she*) couldn't touch (*his/her*) mind, if (*he/she*) did (*his/her*) composure would shatter

(*he'd/she'd*) been alone too long

(*he/she*) wasn't a hormone crazed teenager anymore

her mind went right to the memory of him brown and bare as the day he was born

(*his/her*) death would serve to warn the others

(*his/her*) desire was to be with (*him/her*) and to enjoy the camaraderie they usually shared

(*his/her*) gut said (*he/she*) was capable of more real passion than (*he/she*) was showing (*him/her*)

(*his/her*) idle fantasies hadn't even begun to match the reality

just the thought of (*his/her*) hands on (*his/her*) body gave (*him/her*) more sexual awareness than (*he'd/she'd*) had in months

lived a life of pampered, luxurious excess

never gotten over (*him/her*), and (*he/she*) couldn't stop thinking here was a second chance

often felt as if (*he'd/she'd*) come too close to a lightning bolt

she'd seen naked men before, but never one so remarkably built or remarkably aroused

so far he'd been a total gentleman with her

the (*man/woman*) could give a (*man/woman*) all kinds of fantasies with that wicked smile alone

the thought brought (*him/her*) to (*his/her*) knees

the thought of him making love to her with his tough, sinewy body, did strange things to her insides

though (*he/she*) was smiling, (*he/she*) saw trouble in (*his/her*) eyes

was everything (*he'd/she'd*) ever imagined and more than (*he'd/she'd*) dreamed

was guilty of many sins and a few crimes

was it obvious (*he/she*) had a fervent wish

why did (*men/women*) always go there—searching for answers to questions they really didn't want to hear

with a flicker of worry (*he/she*) kept the thought to (*himself/herself*)

wondered what his rough hands would feel like against her skin

worked long and hard to gain credibility

Questions

♥~♥

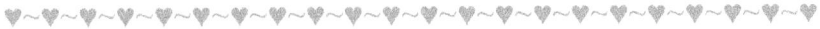

could he enjoy her physically without allowing himself to fall back into the emotional trap

could she bear to see rage and disgust in his eyes when he looked at her

didn't know what she had accomplished by refusing him

didn't know what to think

had thousands of questions to ask

his brows knit slightly, making her wonder what he found perplexing about her question

how had (*he/she*) known (*he/she*) hungered for intimacy that went beyond sex

impulsive action had carried (*him/her*) this far, but was it salvation or disaster

needed to keep an open mind

now what was she supposed to do—stay away from him after he fired every nerve in her body?

seemed strangely preoccupied by something

she'd be a fool to trust a man to whom everyone was merely a tool to be used and discarded

she'd thought they were going to make love

was (*he/she*) repeating the same mistake (*he'd/she'd*) made her whole life

was there a chance (*he/she*) could salvage the relationship?

wasn't sure (*he/she*) wanted to go back to the cutthroat world of large law firms

wasn't sure if (*he/she*) were relieved or annoyed

what would it be like if (*he/she*) kissed (*him/her*) (*in/with*) (*real/genuine*) passion

where in the world had (*he/she*) learned to dance like that

where were they supposed to go from here

while (*he/she*) waited for (*his/her*) response, (*his/her*) heart raced with anxiety

why couldn't (*he/she*) have left well enough alone

why did all of (*his/her*) senses seem suddenly heightened when (*he/she*) was around (*him/her*)

why had (*he/she*) come back and opened all these old wounds

wondered if (*he/she*) regretted the choice (*he'd/she'd*) made all those years ago

wondered why (*he'd/she'd*) come all this way, and how soon (*he/she*) could leave

would (*he/she*) let what was simmering between them grow into something more would (*he/she*) survive if (*he/she*) surrendered to the craving (*he/she*) saw in the smoldering depths of (*his/her*) eyes

Acknowledgment

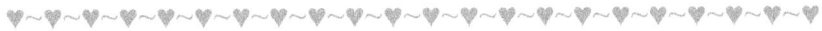

❤~❤~❤~❤~❤~❤~❤~❤~❤~❤~❤~❤~❤~❤~❤~❤~❤~❤~❤~❤

a fragile, needy woman who hadn't been able to take care of herself

a (*man/woman*) who knew how to care, even if (*he/she*) didn't allow (*himself/herself*) to do it

a (*man/woman*) with (*his/her*) own mind

air was thick with unspoken emotions

all (*he/she*) could do was treasure the time they had together

amazing how an incident in (*his/her*) life that had happened so long ago could come back to haunt (*him/her*)

closing (*his/her*) eyes, (*he/she*) knew (*he/she*) had to push (*him/her*) away

coaxing her into bed was the exact antidote he needed to forget about being betrayed

could so easily give in to the whispers of temptation

every kill brought him closer to the edge of madness

every part of his soul screamed for him to hold her by his side

exactly the sort of place where (*he/she*) could ratchet up their relationship to the next level

fate had changed (*his/her*) life

for the first time in weeks the gnawing ache inside (*him/her*) eased

had a right to some anger, some hurt and some answers

had to admit, if only to (*himself/herself*), that the past was never very far away

(*he/she*) did things to (*him/her*)—made (*him/her*) feel things (*he'd/she'd*) never felt for another (*man/woman*) (*he/she*) hadn't known it was possible to love someone so deeply, so completely, in such a short time

he'd pushed her too far, too quickly

(*he'd/she'd*) try not to hurt (*him/her*) when it was time to go

(*he/she*) was the sort who deserved a forever kind of (*man/woman*)

(*his/her*) whole life was unraveling around (*him/her*), and no matter what (*he/she*) did, (*he/she*) couldn't seem to hold it all together

(*his/her*) looks had brought (*him/her*) nothing but trouble

how little (*he/she*) really knew (*him/her*) hit (*him/her*) squarely between the eyes

how simple it would be to slide into a physical relationship

if (*he/she*) let (*him/her*), (*he'd/she'd*) love (*him/her*) and leave (*him/her*) like everyone else did

it was (*his/her*) gift and (*his/her*) curse that (*he/she*) would feel too much

it wasn't the first time (*he'd/she'd*) tried to enchant (*him/her*)

knew (*his/her*) instincts would be to confront and overcome

loving (*him/her*) physically could only lead to loving (*him/her*) emotionally

made the mistake of meeting (*his/her*) eyes and the burn of heat in their deeply shadowed depths

never noticed before what a perfect mouth (*he/she*) had

no match for his immense strength

now (*he/she*) was insulting (*his/her*) intellect

realized he'd balled his hand into a tight fist

reliability and responsibility hadn't been his strong points

scared (*him/her*) how much (*he/she*) was coming to mean to (*him/her*)

she couldn't do anything to control the chemical reactions in her body

she'd known this moment would arrive. No lie lasted forever

she had no relatives, no boyfriend—that made her the perfect (*agent/target*)

she made something inside him pay attention to things he hadn't let himself feel in a long time

she realized her attitude toward sex had changed; if approached, she wanted what he offered

she'd buried her dreams, surrendered her innocence

short-term benefits of sex could cure what ailed you

swallowed back (*his/her*) last lingering doubt

the more time (*he/she*) spent with (*him/her*) the harder it was going to be to leave

the realization (*he/she*) was still crippled by that memory came as a shock

the wall (*he'd/she'd*) spent so many years erecting and fortifying shattered

the weight of (*his/her*) beliefs crashed down on (*him/her*)

the (*man/woman*) awakened something in (*him/her*) that hadn't been touched in years

there was no denying (*he/she*) would make the perfect political (*husband/wife*)

there were precious few things (*he/she*) would be able to take with (*him/her*)

was buck naked under (*his/the*) sheets

was going to be a challenge sharing (*himself/herself*) and (*his/her*) life with a (*husband/wife*)

when (*his/her*) arms closed around (*him/her*), it felt like (*he'd/she'd*) come home

whether (*he/she*) wanted to admit it or not, (*he/she*) was wildly attracted to...

Memories

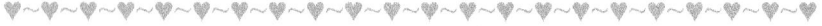

all her life she'd heard she was built for breeding

as he'd last seen her drifted through his thoughts and rubbed every edge of his conscience

for this moment he wanted to enjoy the woman he remembered

had damaged her confidence and scarred her

hadn't seen (*him/her*) this vulnerable since...

(*he'd/she'd*) come back to the town (*he'd/she'd*) left behind forever

her body remembered the sound of his voice

his gut kicked as his body reacted to the memory of them together

(*his/her*) thoughts pulled (*him/her*) back to a faded, but never forgotten memory

it was her glorious hair that had first attracted him to her

knew every expression of (*his/her*) face

reminding (*him/her*) at every turn how much (*he'd/she'd*) given up

she caught a hint of his aftershave and a whole lot of unwanted memories

she was remembering the way he'd made love to her, the way her body responded to his very touch

sifting through the memories of every moment (*he'd/she'd*) spent with (*him/her*)

smoky images haunted (*his/her*) memories, hung on the edge of recall

snorted with self-disgust

someday (*he'd/she'd*) be able to smell (*his/her*) (*cologne/ perfume*) without remembering (*his/her*) touch

taunting (*him/her*) with thoughts of what might have been

the flash was so strong, for a fractured second (*he/she*) was thrown back in time

the memories were as clear and crisp as they'd been the moment the pictures had been taken

the women in his family were adored and treasured by the men

they were both reminded of the first time they'd made love

years ago she'd left, a foolish girl who couldn't conceive of a universe that didn't revolve around her

Five Senses

Sight

♥~♥

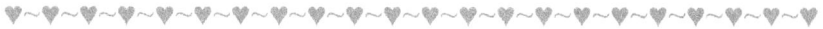

admire	behold	catch a glimpse
display	glance	inspect
look at	notice	observe
picture	scan	scene
see	spy upon	stare
view	vision	vista
watch		

a single tear rolled down her cheek, moonlight catching it and making it shine

black slacks and a snug fitting T-shirt

could see the curve of her cheek, the shape of her lips in the slant of moonlight

did a quick scan of the interior with his night vision goggles

fine tuned the focus on his binoculars

held in thrall by the woman whose eyes had mesmerized him

her face was too pale, her eyes too wide

his impressive body lit only by a hazy moon

(*his/her*) damp jeans fit (*him/her*) perfectly

let her gaze wander down the cleft in his spine, past the smooth curve of his waist

made a quick visual sweep of the room

noticed the way his wet T-shirt sculpted over the muscles of his arms and chest opened (*his/her*) eyes as sunlight streamed through the windows, warming (*him/her*)

she was what every man dreamed of touching

shut (*his/her*) eyes and gave (*himself/herself*) over to feeling

soaked shirt clinging to the hard planes of his torso

stared across the room, she'd forgotten how good looking he was

stared at his physique and his behind in the skin-tight jeans

stood there like a fallen (*god/goddess*), drenched in moonlight

sun turned (*his/her*) hair to copper

the (*black/beige*) trench coat swirled as he jumped to the sidewalk

the first time (*he'd/she'd*) looked into (*his/her*) eyes he'd felt like (*he'd/she'd*) been zapped by . . .

the light cast tricky shadows across his darkly stubbled face

the look in (*his/her*) eyes was wild

the lusciousness of her full lips had his gaze returning to her face

the (*man/woman*) was something incredible to look at

the rain (*plastered/pelted*) (*his/her*) hair to (*his/her*) head

the shadow of her dark nipples against the fabric

visions of wild, raging sex had (*his/her*) head spinning

watched (*his/her*) backside with appreciation

watched the (*man/woman*) step into the elevator the doors quietly swishing shut

when she lifted her arms her shirt rose, giving him a glimpse of tanned skin

Smell

♥~♥

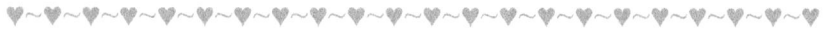

aroma	body spray	bouquet
cologne	dirty	earthy
essence	fetid	fishy
flowery	fragrance	fresh
get a whiff of	mildewed	moist
moldy	musty	nauseating
odor	perfume(*d*)	pungent
putrid	reek	rotten
scent	skunky	sniff
spicy	sour	spoiled
stench	stink	sweaty
sweet	tang	tart

a gentle breeze drifted past, carrying the subtle scent of roses

achingly familiar aroma of incense and musk

acrid smell of smoke

air smelled like rotting garbage

beneath the rich scent of blood were other scents

caught the drift of her scent, part woman, part leather, part something else

closing (*his/her*) eyes, (*he/she*) breathed deeply

cloying scent of roses in the still air made her stomach churn

comforting scent of sausage and bacon frying

coppery smell of violence slapped (*him/her*) in the face

could smell her, a soft, pretty fragrance that seemed to whisper in his ear

could smell her hair fresh, clean with sexy undertones

could taste him on her lips, simply by catching his scent

delicate scents drifted up

edged close enough to inhale the fragrant softness of her skin and hair

eyes watered from the stench

her (*pheromones/scent*) were clouding his (*head/thoughts/ concentration/judgment*)

(*he/she*) caught the drift of (*his/her*) scent, part (*man/woman*), part leather, part something else

(*he/she*) inhaled, dragging (*his/her*) scent deep into (*his/her*) lungs

(*he/she*) smelled like soap, shampoo and (*man/woman*)

(*he/she*) wore a heavy dose of (*aftershave/perfume*)

(*her/his*) scent curled through (*his/her*) memory

(*her/his*) scent lingered like poison on (*his/her*) sheets

(*her/his*) scent surrounded (*him/her*), a blend of soap, toothpaste and cologne

(*her/his*) senses filled with (*his/her*) scent

his clean, male smell filled her nostrils and made her lightheaded

his clean, spicy scent invaded her head and weakened her knees

his cologne, a dark, rich fragrance

his earthy scent bloomed in her nostrils

his scent, some expensive outdoor cologne, wafted between them

inhaled the scent of sand and seaweed

inhaling the essence of the woman

inhaling the scent of warm spice and male heat

more subtle, was her own unique hot scent

never smelled anything like her clean rose-scented flesh

nostrils flaring as (*he/she*) inhaled

noxious scent of unwashed flesh

room was heavy with the rich aroma of lust and sex

scent of excrement, sweat and fear

scent of (*his/her*) hair

scent of leather and silk

scent of night-blooming flowers

scent of wood smoke and wet leaves

she enveloped him in a drift of exotic perfume

smelled like flowers and sunshine

smelled like the lava soap he'd used to wash with

soft, subtle, vanilla and something exotic

sour smell of his breath hit her like a slap

spicy, masculine scent of him

spicy smell of beef stew and chili-peppers

steam rising from (*his/her*) cup smelled like heaven

strong smell of horses and hay

sweet scent of grain and leather

sweetness of her breath

the breeze shifted and her scent, hot sultry and compelling filled him

the engine still running, (*he/she*) could smell the gasoline exhaust

the faint feminine scent of her perfume drifted into his senses

the fruity scent of antibacterial soap tingled (*his/her*) nose

the grass smelled strong and sweet

the rich earthy scent of dew, damp grass and flowering trees

the room oozed with the sweet floral perfume

the scent of cheap scotch

the scent of grilling hot dogs

the scent of his cologne traveled along her nerve endings

the smell of blood hit (*his/her*) system like a shot of adrenaline

the smell of human desperation

the smell of old, rotting flesh and vomit

the smell of ozone and rain mixing with the sharper smell of fear

the smell of sex lingered in the air

the smell of tobacco

the stink of mildew and decay hung heavy in the damp air

the sweet smell of (*rain/musty wet ground/earthy leaves/ mud*) assailed her

the tempting sweetness of incense clung to her skin

the unique scent of her skin and hair, the female essence of the woman

thick smell of blood and sweaty humanity

warm, (*masculine/leather/woodsy*) scent

Create Your Own Tags!!!

Taste

♥~♥~♥~♥~♥~♥~♥~♥~♥~♥~♥~♥~♥~♥~♥~♥~♥~♥~♥

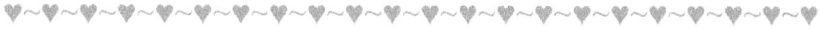

bite	bite into	chew
crunch	drink	eat
essence	flavor	gnaw
kick	lave	lick
morsel	mouthful	nibble
nip	piquancy	ravish
sample	savor	season
sip	spiciness	swallow
tang	tartness	taste
test	try	zest

chocolate melted on (*his/her*) tongue

couldn't believe how good (*he/she*) tasted

flavor exploded in (*his/her*) mouth

had never sampled anything sweeter than the honey of her mouth

he loved the flavor of her, the quietly seductive taste that clung to her skin

her mouth was sweet and damp, her tongue stroking against his

his mouth was filled with the taste of her

mouth felt full of cotton

savoring (*his/her*) delicious mouth

she tasted better than anything he could remember

she tasted of heat and cinnamon

she tasted of wicked temptation and sinful delights

she tasted the sweet tartness of her own blood on his lips

still had the taste of (*him/her*) in (*his/her*) mouth

sweet-musky, feminine, he'd forgotten how good a woman could taste

tasted dark and dangerous

tasted like everything (*he'd/she'd*) ever wanted

tasted like sweetened coffee/passion too long denied

tasted of the (*strawberries/any food*) they'd had for dinner

the blend of sweet Texas onion and crispy coating melted on (*his/her*) tongue

the faintly salty taste of (*his/her*) own blood

the taste of (*him/her*) was addictive

was sweet as wild honey

Touch

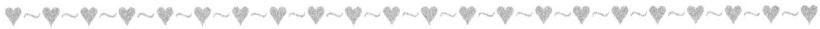

bite	blow	brush
bump	burrow	bury
buss	caress	circle
claw	clutch	collide
come together	contact	converge
cover	creep	crush
cuddle	cup	curl
drag	draw	embrace
feel	feel up	fiddle with
finger	flick	flit
fondle	frisk	fumble
glance	glide	grind
grip	graze	grope
handle	hit	hold
huddle	hug	impact

join	kiss	knead
lap	lay a hand on	link with
maneuver	manhandle	mash
massage	mold	muzzle
neck	nestle	nuzzle
nudge	outline	palm
partake	pat	paw
peck	pet	pinch
press	probe	pull
push	rasp	reach
rim	run	rub
scrape	scratch	scrub
shave	shift	skim
slide	smack	smooth
snuggle	solid and hard	soothe
spank	splay	spread
squeeze	stretch	strike
stroke	suck	sweep
swipe	tangle	tap
taste	tease	thumb
thump	tickle	tip
tongue	touching	toy
trace	trail	tug
tunnel	twiddle	twirl
twist	work	wrap

a hand smoothed his brow with the infinite care of a mother's touch

a strong, heavy heartbeat thumped against (*his/her*) fingertips absently testing the pulse at the base of (*his/her*) neck

body tingled with awareness

closed (*his/her*) eyes and savored the exquisite feel of (*him/her*)

cool morning air whispered across the heated flush of (*his/her*) body

could almost feel his fingers on her skin just by the look in his eyes

could feel the weight of (*his/her*) burning gaze on (*his/her*) skin

delighted in the sensation of (*his/her*) hand in (*his/hers*)

felt like hot silk in his arms

felt the bunching and quivering of a muscle beneath her hand

felt the tiny beads of sweat across (*his/her*) brow

fingers brushed (*his/her*) cheek

fingers lingering a moment to caress her small, neat handwriting

fingers skimmed up her stomach, sending quivers of anticipation

fingers toyed with the top button of his pants

fingertips sculpting the curve of (*his/her*) cheek and the line of (*his/her*) jaw

fingertips trailed down the side of (*his/her*) face

gently (*touched/pressed/probed*) (*his/ her*) throbbing cheek and wished (*he/she*) didn't have a headache

gingerly fingered the photograph

hand came to rest at (*his/her*) waist

he half growled, half laughed and pulled her even closer

he'd made certain they were connected the entire afternoon

(*he/she*) cradled the side of (*his/her*) cheek

(*he/she*) held the baggie of crushed ice to (*his/her*) (*face/cheek/eye/head*) her cheek throbbed and she gently touched it

her hands moved up and down his back in a searching motion

her neck was warm satin beneath his stroking fingers

her skin felt as baby soft as he remembered

her skin was remarkably warm through her blouse

her soft exhalation floated across his mouth

his calloused hands were rough on her sensitive skin

his finger halted her moving lips, the touch firm and gentle

(*his/her*) touch a feather-light caress

intimately he pulled her against him until their lower bodies swayed in unison

lay a hand on

lifted one hand and smoothed (*his/her*) hair back from (*his/her*) face

lifting (*his/her*) face to the moist wind

lips brushing the edge of her ear, sending shivers rippling up her spine

loved the way (*his/her*) hair felt between (*his/her*) fingers

marveled at her softness

ran a finger down the hard planes of his chest

reached out slowly to weave (*his/her*) fingers through (*his/her*) hair

reverently touched the marks on (*his/her*) flesh with the tips of (*his/her*) fingers

she dared to put her hand on his chest, felt the rapid beat of his heart

she found the brush of his evening beard against the softness of her skin sexy

she placed her hand in his and let him wind their way to the dance floor

shivered at the touch of (*his/her*) skin on (*his/hers*)

skin felt warm and tingly

skin was warm and (*he/she*) could feel calluses on (*his/her*) palms and fingers

slightly rough textured touch

smoothed her hair, enjoying the texture of it under his palm

stroking the dark circle under one eye with the pad of his thumb

sultry heat (*he/she*) was giving off

talented mouth and even more talented hands

the grass beneath (*him/her*) soft and inviting

the heat of (*him/her*) flowed through (*him/her*), lashing (*his/her*) skin and stirring the hunger

the mere touch of (*his/her*) hand made (*his/her*) skin tingle

the slight shiver from (*his/her*) touch made (*him/her*) pause

tipped her chin up with his fingers

took his hand and felt the warm, rough texture against her skin

touch burned through the cotton of (*his/her*) knit sweater

toyed with her fragile fingers

tracing the scars across the backs of his knuckles

wanted to touch his mouth, to run her fingers over the full lips to test their softness

wondering if his skin would be warm to her touch

Hearing

♥~♥

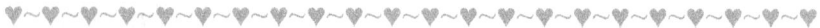

bang	blare	blast
boom	buzz	clamor
clank	clatter	clink
crash	echo	hear
hiss	hum	jingle
listen	purr	racket
rattle	refrain	reverberation
ricochet	ring	rustle
silence	song	swish
tinkle	thud	tune
whine	whisper	whistle
whoosh		

Additional Extras

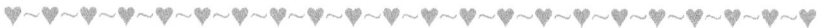

♥~♥

bellow	call out	exclaim
holler	roar	scream
shriek	yell	yelp

a whisper of movement

an ache in his voice

cane made a thumping sound on the hardwood floor

chatter of insects in the grass

cleaned the fork with a satisfied purr

could hear the faint sounds of the rotors in the distance

could hear the satisfying smack of wood against bone

couldn't hear anything beyond the noise of the fire

couldn't hear over the roar of the chopper blades

cowboy boots that echoed on the (*hardwood/wooden*) floor

crystal earrings made a tinkling sound that floated on the air

gentle whoosh of the sea on the (*rocks/shore*)

heard her sigh, the sound soft as the slow fall of rain

heard nothing but the roar and pump of (*his/her*) heartbeat

her jacket brushed against his, a soft shush of fabric against fabric

(*his/her*) laugh low, musical

(*his/her*) voice, velvet seduction, black magic

hypnotic sound of water lapping against rock

listened to the strum of (*his/her*) heart

no mistaking the hungry, sensual growl low in his throat

she shifted restlessly, her movements a faint whisper of silk against cotton

she'd never known her own name could sound so sexy

small, insistent voice at the back of his mind warned him to stop

sultry, sensuous things (*he/she*) whispered to (*him/her*) in the dark

the angry clicks her heels made on the tile floor as she marched down the hallway

the heels of her boots echoed throughout the silence of the concrete parking area

the intimate feel of (*his/her*) voice

the music filled the air with sensual and erotic melodies

the roar of the chopper was unmistakable

there was the sound of a slap

whispered softly in (*his/her*) ear

Passion

Attraction, Desire

♥~♥

a crackle of energy passed between them, hot and raw, carnal

acute awareness of stunning male power and strength

a deep, sexual hunger stirred to life in his mid-section

a distinct warmth flooded the area between her legs

a gush of feminine awareness

a hot blush crept over her (*neck and face/whole body*)

a jolt of sexual energy that rocked him to the bone

a little ball of need burst to life at the pit of her stomach

a low moan slipped past her lips, a husky helpless sound of want

a primitive force inside him that demanded he reach for her

a rare sexual aura

a spike of heat caught (*him/her*) low in the gut

all he could do to keep from dragging her down onto his lap

already secretly noted how he filled out his jeans

an explosion of pleasure and need went off inside (*him/her*)

anticipation thickened the air in (*his/her*) lungs

appeasing her sexual hunger was going to be his pleasure

aroused her as no man ever had

aware of her all along his length

aware of her in every pore of his body—her nearness, the scent of her, the heat of her skin

awareness filled (*his/her*) every pore, even the air (*he/she*) breathed

beat of forbidden desire, strong, thick and unrelenting

blood in (*his/her*) veins went hot and molten

body was long and hard and muscular

breath caught on a surge of yearning so abrupt and intense it felt like pain

breath wobbled, catching in a sexual way

buried his face in the hollow of her throat where he could drink in her scent

buried long fingers in the wet tangle of (*his/her*) hair

caught her hand and pressed it to the bulge in his zipper

closed her eyes on a moan when he caught the lobe of her ear between his teeth

coiling arousal in her core

conscious that (*he/she*) was staring, (*he/she*) dragged (*his/her*) gaze back up to (*his/her*) face

could barely remember his name past the pounding pulse (*in his crotch/of his erection*)

could have floated on this whisper thin cloud of sensation forever

could no longer ignore the delicious heat of carnal attraction

couldn't remember ever feeling this tight with need

cradled (*his/her*) face in his hands and closed (*his/her*) eyes

dark heat in (*his/her*) eyes

deep in the center of (*his/her*) being was a hungry throb that didn't want to be denied

desire a pulsing, throbbing need that made him rock hard

desire clawed at (*him/her*), hot and sharp

desire lit up his (*blue/gray/hazel*) eyes

desire made (*him/her*) feel faint

desire twisting (*his/her*) guts and adding to (*his/her*) ache

didn't pause to ask (*himself/herself*) if (*he/she*) was ready for the needs (*he/she*) read in (*his/her*) eyes

didn't want to cross over any lines (*he'd/she'd*) regret

driven by (*his/her*) own needs, (*he/she*) pulled at (*his/her*) shirt

each caress subtly urging her closer and closer to him

every hormone in her body sizzled

every touch tingled as though (*he/she*) were holding a live wire

everywhere she touched him he burned – (*chest/belly/thighs*)

eyes met with a force that licked through (*his/her*) body

felt an arrow of liquid heat shoot straight to (*his/her*) groin

felt as though (*he/she*) were burning alive from the inside out

felt her muscles tighten as desire warmed (*him/her*) to the core

felt her shyness in the way she hesitated, in her awkward movements

felt the wonder of (*him/her*) in every pore, every nerve, with every pulse

flare of response in (*his/her*) body

fresh urgency plowed through (*him/her*) when (*he/she*) pressed against (*him/her*)

frissons of fire and ice raced up (*his/her*) spine

frustrated and hungry for him, she crossed her legs

glance drifted over his open shirt, bare chest and shoeless feet

gliding her hands up his sexy, sculpted abdomen

grazing his jaw against her ear, he growled low in his throat

had a body to die for and he was slowly drawing his last breath

hadn't counted on taking one look at her and getting slammed in the chest with what felt like a (*hammer/sledge*) blow

in his arms she felt small, feminine and safe

hands were straying, skimming downward toward places that
didn't need any attention right now

hard hum of lust in (*his/her*) veins

he felt tight and hot, his body making urgent demands

he made her heart do handsprings in her chest

(*he/she*) groaned in raw appreciation

(*he/she*) was in every dream, every waking thought

heart skipped, then started to race

heat curled inside (*him/her*), threatening (*his/her*) control

heat in (*his/her*) veins and between (*his/her*) legs

heightened beat of (*his/her*) pulse

her aura washed him with heat and desire

her body throbbed in areas she'd never known a body could
throb

her body warmed under his regard, aching for his touch

her gaze drifted over him, his body heating with each lingering
visual caress

her gaze snared with his and her pulse flickered and leaped

her hips flowed into his, their bodies intimately and perfectly
aligned to each other

her lips presented a temptation that made him edgy

her nerves danced, her brain raced, and her stomach did a
quick somersault

her womb contracted with need at the sight of him

his body hardened at the thought of spending the night with her

(*his/her*) body's most primal reaction kicked in with a
vengeance

(*his/her*) brain didn't know what to do, but (*his/her*) body did

his brain faltered when her scent enveloped him

his breath hot on her ear as he nibbled her lobe

his calloused hands caressed as his mouth promised rapture

his gaze locked with hers with a powerful slam of something hot and steamy

his hands were on her body, hard and masculine

(*his/her*) body practically convulsed with sexual energy

(*his/her*) eyes closed

his lips brushed over her ear and made her shiver

his muscular power surrounded her

his palm skimmed around to the front, fingertips slipping across the lace top of her stocking

his pulse kicked, an instant response to the sensations that swamped his body

hot spark of reaction in (*his/her*) eyes

huge, swollen bulge, cupped by the soft worn fabric

if he touched her she'd incinerate, and if he didn't, she'd die

if there had been any doubt of his need before, there certainly was none now

inch by inch she gradually relaxed beneath him

(*instant/fierce/intense/savage*) desire made him draw a harsh, ragged breath

jeans and boxers fell to his ankles with a whoosh

knew the shape and fullness of her lips

knowledge flashed in her eyes, grabbed him by the throat

lightheaded and breathing hard (*he/she*) clenched (*his/her*) fists at (*his/her*) sides to keep from (*rushing/pulling*) (*her/him*) into (*his/her*) arms

lit a powder keg in (*his/her*) gut

logic replaced by a visceral curl of appreciation

looking at (*him/her*) as if nothing else in the world mattered

moistened cherry red lips with a suggestive sweep of her tongue moisture gathered thickly between her thighs

naked desire warmed the dazed expression in (*his/her*) eyes

nearly overcome, (*he/she*) groaned

need began to consume (*him/her*) like a flame sucking up oxygen

need hammered at (*his/her*) common sense

never felt such primal attraction to any (*male/man*) before

no man had ever made her skin tingle just by looking at her

nothing on earth could have kept him from tasting her sweet, rosy lips

paused to tame his rapid breathing and heartbeat

picked her up and carried her to his bed

recognized the ragged heat, the sweet pull of desire

restless, faintly impatient and a little rough

restless throb of desire in her veins

riding the fine edge between not enough and almost too much

rush of desire that clawed and clutched at his insides

seductive whisper stroked over (*him/her*) with the effect of a soft, warm kiss

sensations (*he'd/she'd*) never before experienced

sexual excitement curled in (*his/her*) stomach

sexual vibes were pouring off (*him/her*)

(*he/she*) wanted (*him/her*) with a ferocity that terrified (*him/her*)

she was drowning in man, in the taste and scent and feel of him

sinfully erotic movement of (*his/her*) hips

slipping her arms around his magnificent muscled back

slow roll in her stomach, the tripping of her pulse

stared into one another's heavy-lidded eyes

stared at her soft body, lush with curves and ripe with passion

stared at the carpet beneath (*his/her*) feet and tried to form complete sentences

stared at the pulse throbbing in the base of his strong throat

still ached for the promise in (*his/her*) eyes of things to come

stirred (*his/her*) libido in all kinds of forbidden ways

subtly shifting so the hot, hard ridge of his erection was cradled snugly between her thighs

supported (*his/her*) weight carefully on (*his/her*) elbow

surrendered to the restlessness inside (*him/her*)

temptation rocked through (*his/her*) veins

tension thickened the blood in (*his/her*) veins

the air shimmered around them, grew taut

the blaze of desire that filled (*his/her*) eyes transfixed (*him/her*)

the feel of her soft curves, and long lines

the force of his aura crashed through her like a tidal wave, leaving her wet and ready

the intensity and immediacy of attraction mystified her

the little purr that sounded in her throat enticed him to draw the kiss out

the man was a walking hormone

the restless desire in (*his/her*) eyes had (*his/her*) heart racing

the restraint and control (*he'd/she'd*) tried holding on to was slowly loosening

the sexual tension was a constant undercurrent

the torture of wanting (*him/her*) was so great (*he/she*) could hardly stand it

thick beat of awareness in (*his/her*) blood

those long forgotten needs had been awakened

throbbing desire rolled into one slow roll of want

to feel her heat and taste the texture of her skin

to inhale the scent of (*him/her*)

traitorous heart turned over at just (*his/her*) smile

tugged at (*his/her*) (*shirt/blouse*), worked (*his/her*) hands beneath it

waited with every nerve in (*his/her*) body humming taut

wanted (*him/her*) desperately, with a sudden fierce longing that almost knocked (*him/her*) off his feet

when she met his gaze, he felt an involuntary tightening low in his gut

with a sigh she settled in his arms, her cheek against his chest

Hugging, Touching

♥~♥

a gentle shift, body to body

arched her back, impatient with the barrier of her bra

big, dark hand tugging at the faded denim

brushed her fingers over his collar and the ends of his hair

caressed her with an unexpected tenderness

caressed the line of her back down to the first hint of her buttocks

clung to him as if he were her lifeline

clung to his shoulders

(*dipped/drove/eased/plunged*) his finger(s) inside her

dusting her rigid nipples across his chest

eased his shirt off, running her hands over his chest

felt every curve, every line of her body as if it were on fire

fingers speared into the silky strands of her hair

fingers traced the subtle shape of each dip and turn

flat on her back beneath his damp, powerful body

gave (*him/her*) a swift hug

gripped her chin in his big hand, tilting her face upward

he held her length pressed to his

he nudged her hips forward, right up against him

he swayed her into a dance

heart beating hard against her palm

held (*his/her*) face, tracing the bones with (*his/her*) fingertips

(*his/her*) caressing hands stilled on (*his/her*) back

his expert touch brought every nerve ending brutally to life

his finger stroked up her ribs, to the edge of her bra

his finger traced her (*breast/nipple/mouth*)

his hand skimmed down her back, rested on her hip

his hands centered at her waist

his hands coaxed and caressed her

his large hands circled her wrist, held her captive

his touch awakened an aching hunger deep within her womb

languid, swirling strokes up and down her back

leaned into (*his/her*) embrace

levering (*himself/herself*) up on (*his/her*) elbow, (*he/she*) traced the shape of (*his/her*) face with (*his/her*) finger

lifted (*his/her*) palm to (*his/her*) lips

moaning, (*he/she*) grabbed (*his/her*) shoulders

molded that rock hard body to hers

pressed tightly together, his (*cock/member/etc.*) throbbed, and his body still thought sex was the best answer

pushing the fabric aside to touch the underside of her breast

ran a warm, smooth hand down (*his/her*) back

rubbed the (*thick ridge/hard length of his erection*)

running the palm of (*his/her*) hand up and down the length of (*his/her*) body

skin sizzled where (*he/she*) pressed against (*him/her*)

sliding one hand up beneath the hem of her shirt, needing to feel the smooth sweep of her skin against his

slipped a (*finger/hand*) beneath her (*chin/neck*)

slowly, lingeringly traced a path from her bottom to her breasts

spread (*his/her*) fingers through (*his/her*) hair and arched closer

stroked her (*neck/cheek/face*)

strong competent hand roaming her body

swallowed harshly as (*his/her*) hand touched (*his/her*) skin

the elegant indention of her spine drew his fingertips

the touch and taste of (*him/her*) filled (*him/her*) with emotions and sensations (*he/she*) hadn't known in years

the world shifted beneath his feet when she fell against him

thumbs stroked (*his/her*) cheekbones

took her hand and (*put it on his heart/drew her close*)

wasn't sure where he began and she left off

with her hands on his chest, she felt his heart pounding wildly beneath his skin

Motion & Undressing

♥~♥

before she lost her nerve, she pushed him to his back and climbed astride him

cupped her hips and pulled her close

eased her onto the (*bed/floor/desk/stairs*)

gently grinding himself against her

grabbed the (*edge/bottom*) of her tank top and pulled the cotton up and over her

gripped her hips and dragged her to the edge of the mattress, then dropped to his knees on the floor

had (*him/her*) flat on (*his/her*) back/ lowered her to the bed

he eased onto the bed crawling over her on all fours

(*he/she*) reached for the hem of (*his/her*) t-shirt, (*he/she*) lifted (his/her) arms and let (*him/her*) pull the cotton up and over (*his/her*) head

hooked his fingers in the edge of her panties, gave one easy tug

lost in her in the moment, he backed her against the...(*yard, barn, room*)

moonlight filled the room with an ethereal light that bathed her flawless skin as he stretched her out on the sheets

picked her up and carried her (*back/to*) bed

pinned her beneath his hard, aching body

pinning her to the (*bed/table/couch/wall*) with gentle finesse

popping the button on her jeans she shimmied the ultra-tight denim down her long legs and stepped free

pulling away long enough to shuck his jeans and briefs

quickly he rolled away to the bedside table, grabbing the condoms he'd bought

rolling in a heated slide of skin against skin

she reached for the hem of his t-shirt, he lifted his arms and let her pull the cotton up and over his head

she stepped closer, knowing what she would find. His huge arousal hit her hip

she twined her arms around his neck, hooked her ankles together behind his back

shoving his jeans and underwear down, he kicked them aside and joined her on the bed

stunned by the force of the need pulsating through his blood, he carried her to . . .

sweeping her into his arms, he headed up stairs, down the hall to her bedroom

tightened his hold on her, reluctant to set her down

turned back the covers and nodded toward the bed, then slowly pulled his shirt over his head

with a growl he rolled her onto her back

with her fingers gripping the sheets beside her hips, she rose to him

with swift hands and quick catches of breath, they shed the rest of their clothes

wrestling with a tangle of clothing until they were both naked

Breasts

♥~♥

brush	caress	cup
envelop	grasp/grip	graze
knead	roll	velvety

Nipples

♥~♥

abrade	bite	bud
capture	caress	circle
coiled	curling(*ed*)	dance
devour	drag	draw
engorge	feast	flick
lap	lave	lick
nibble	nip	nuzzle
pearl	pinch	pleasure
probe	prod	rake
rasp	roll	savor(*ing/ed*)
scorch	scrape	squeeze
stab	stroke	suck
surround	swirl	tantalize
taste	taut	tease
thrust	tighten	torment
torture	trace	tug
tweak	worship	wrap(*ped*)

Color

♥~♥

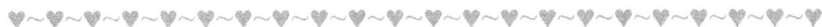

blush	berry	caramel
cherry	coral	dark/dusky
peach	rosy hued	sweet pink

a beautiful soft breast that he glimpsed briefly

a (*wide/warm/hot/large/calloused*) hand cupped her breast and her breath caught in her throat

breasts swollen from her pregnancy spilled heavily into his palms

breasts were small, but perfectly shaped, her nipples flushed dark

buried his nose in the valley between her breasts

burying his face in her breasts, drew one nipple at a time into his mouth

caressing a trail down her arm until he cupped her breast, molding her fullness

could see the faint outline of her nipples beneath the dark, thin material

drew his fingertips up the side of her breast

drew on her nipples, sucking, tonguing and teasing

firm, wet mouth closed over one peak

groaned with want as her breasts pushed against the palms of his hands

he scraped his palms over her nipples

her bare breasts tingled as a draft of air moved across them

her breasts grew heavy, weighted with need

her breasts lay soft and full beneath her blouse

her breasts pressed into his chest, sent pleasure so (*intense/ sharp*) it was almost painful through her body

her breasts rose and fell with shuddering, uneven breaths

her breasts tightened as warm heat seared her

her nipples glistening from his mouth

his hot palm cupped the weight

his thumbs scraped lightly over her rigid nipples

licked the sides of her breasts and inhaled deeply the scent of her skin

high round breasts, tipped with small tight nipples

lifted and kneaded her breast

nipples drawn into tight, small points

nipples had hardened from the very first feel of his lips on hers

one of his hands circled around to the front of her body and cupped a breast

prettiest breasts this side of the county line

pulled her on top of him so that her breasts hung heavy in his face

ran his tongue over the sensual path between her breast

shivered and fought for air when his fingers caressed her nipples, tweaking, tugging

the feel of his fingers stroking her breast electrified her

the sensation of his lips on her nipple

thumb and forefinger met and captured the tight burning peak

thumbs circling, slowly, lightly over her nipples

Kisses

♥~♥

forceful	devoured her mouth	kissed her earlobe
lazy	plunder/plundered	ravish
slow	smooth	suck
sweet	taste	urgent
warm	whisper	

a coming home kind of kiss where body parts acclimate themselves to familiar territory

a full contact, wet-tongued, tonsil-probing kiss

a hint of tightly harnessed control

a light teasing kiss, just enough to still her resistance

an unexpected measure of wildness in his taste

bared her skin and scattered tiny love-bites over her shoulder

began a tortuous trail along her jaw line with his tongue and nibbling teeth

brushing his firm, full, sexy lips back and forth over hers

captured his mouth in a kiss that made his head reel

clamping her face with his big hands he captured her mouth in a good morning kiss

crushed his mouth to hers

deepened the pressure with his strong, hard lips

dropped a feather-light kiss on (*his/her*) forehead

every bit as raw and unapologetic as it was seductive

exerted a more provocative pressure with his mouth

exploiting her mouth for all it was worth

eyelids fluttered closed, and on a sigh she gave in to the pleasure he offered

feel the moist heat of (*his/her*) mouth against (*his/hers*)

forceful demand of his mouth

gently sucking her lower lip

gripping a fistful of her short dark curls, he slanted his mouth over hers

groaned beneath his breath, settled his mouth on her lips

groaned when he felt her shudder

growling soft and low in his throat, he dragged his mouth away

had been hungry for the taste of her for days

he kissed her with his entire body, surrounding her as they danced

he paused, drew a ragged breath

he silenced her with a hard kiss

(*he/she*) slid down (*his/her*) body, spreading open-mouthed kisses as (*he/she*) went

heated and uninvited, his mouth on her at last

he made love to her mouth letting her know how he would make love to body

her luscious lips wandered over him, sucking, licking, teasing

her mouth was following the path of her hands—down toward parts of him that ached to have her taste him

her pink lips whispering his name in anxious abandon

(*his/her*) breath whispered over (*his/her*) neck

(*his/her*) hands plunged into (*his/her*) hair, pulling (*his/her*) head closer

(*his/her*) kiss ignited a bone-melting fire that spread through (*his/her*) blood

his kiss lightly chafed his beard across her jaw

(*his/her*) kiss spilled through to (*his/her*) soul

his low growl of approval vibrated into her

(*his/her*) mouth all but consumed (*him/her*) in a rush of frantic kisses

his mouth firm and strong, his lips gentle

his mouth never left hers as he kicked the door closed

his mouth opened on her neck, placing soft, wet, love bites here and there

(*his/her*) tongue rimmed (*his/her*) lips

hot liquid kisses pushed reality to the deepest corners of (*his/her*) mind

kissed her forehead gently, reluctant to release her

kissed her knuckles like a gallant knight of long ago

kissed her ribs, her cleavage, each breast and finally her mouth

kissed her with toe-curling determination

kissed (*him/her*) with all the pent up stress of the past weeks

kissed his clean-shaven cheek

kissed his way to her soft belly while his fingers combed through her (*tight/damp*) curls

kissed like he wanted to devour

kissed so thoroughly and possessively that she wasn't herself

kisses were (*hungry/soft and unhurried*)

leaned forward and in one smooth movement covered her mouth with his own

left a trail of kisses along the edge of her collarbone

lifted (*his/her*) mouth from (*his/hers*)

lifting the hem of her shirt, he bent his head and kissed her belly

lips wandered across her cheekbones, her eyelids, her chin, nuzzled her ear and nipped her neck

lips were silky, pleasantly resilient

long, slow kisses that clouded (his/her) mind

lowered his head his eyes watching her

lowered his mouth (*eagerly/gently/hungrily*) to hers

lowered his head, his lips hovering just above hers

lowering his head to kiss her soundly and quickly on the lips

luscious anticipation and the slow burn of desire curled through her

met (*his/her*) lips in a searing, demanding kiss

mind blowing lip lock

mindless, drugging kisses that left her shaking, breathless and (*begging/yearning*) for more

mouth (*demanding and greedy/hot and hungry*)

mouth moved down her throat, his tongue hot and wet

mouth opened against hers, asking for permission to take more

mouth tasted and nipped along her (*stomach/throat/thigh*)

nipped lightly at her earlobe and made her shudder

nothing could have prepared her for the mind-blowing intensity of his kiss

open mouthed, wet and deep

opened (*his/her*) mouth, eager for the taste and feel of (*his/her*) tongue stroking (*his/hers*)

passion overrode caution

pressed his lips to the sensitive curve between neck and shoulder

placed his mouth against her ear

planted a searing kiss on her mouth

poured everything he was into the kiss

ravishing with lips and teeth and tongue

rocked him in a way he wouldn't have believed

rubbed his open mouth against her throat

savoring all the subtle, sensual variations of (*his/her*) kiss

savoring the taste of (*his/her*) (*kiss/lips*)

sealed his lips over hers, taking possession of her mouth

seduced her with hot, deep glides of his tongue

she moaned into his mouth

slid his hand to the nape of her neck

slowly, lazily, never breaking eye contact, he lowered his mouth

smooth, warm demand of (*his/her*) mouth

soft, sweet breath against (*his/her*) mouth

softness and heat and unspoken promises

starving, he dived deeper into her mouth

sucked her (*lower/bottom*) lip into his mouth, nipped it, then closed his mouth hard over hers

sucking at (*his/her*) mouth, groaning as their tongues scraped together

surged up over her, kissing her like there was no tomorrow

the first hungry swipe of his tongue took her breath away

the kiss of a man who knew exactly what he (*was doing/ wanted*)

the moment his mouth took hers, he felt the invisible threads already binding them tighten

the soft sound of her sigh whispered through him with need and hunger

the sweet urgency of (*his/her*) kiss

the taste of her mouth silky and warm

the warm pressure of (*his/her*) mouth against (*his/her*)

tipping her head back, cradling it in his palm, he claimed her

tongue boldly swept in

touched his lips to her jaw, dragged them to the corner of her mouth

traced the curve of her cheek with his mouth

tracing the shape of her mouth with the tip of his tongue before stealing another kiss

was a dominant kiss, an expert kiss

was lost the second (*his/her*) lips touched (*his/hers*)

wrestling her swollen lips from his

Create Your Own Tags!!!

Lovemaking

Hero

♥~♥~♥~♥~♥~♥~♥~♥~♥~♥~♥~♥~♥~♥~♥~♥~♥~♥~♥

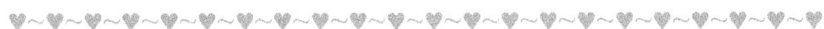

above him her long, slender body curved, she began to rock

acted on pure blind instinct and dark driving need

all he wanted was to feel her naked against him

already thick with blood, more heat rushed to his loins

(*a spike of heat/punch of arousal*) hit him low in the gut

a (*throaty/tender*) (*purr/sigh/gasp*)

backed her up against the wall, capturing her with his hardened body

beneath her panties he caressed damp, downy curls

caught between a sigh and a moan

cupped a hand beneath her bottom, tilted her hips and began a slow rhythm

cupped him in her hand and massaged him until he was rock hard for her

dragged his tongue all the way up her swollen clit

eased himself inside her giving warmth

every cell in (*his/her*) body erupted with need

every roll of his hips was deliberate as he watched her, gauging her response

feeling her body tighten and pulse around him

felt her thighs quiver, her belly (*shudder/tighten*)

felt her body stiffen, breath coming fast and harsh

felt his breath rush out of him as inch by sweet inch she slowly took him into her mouth

fit himself snugly in the (*cradle/vee*) of her thighs

fully aroused, desire pulsing though his swollen and rigid flesh

gently stroking, caressing, fanning the flames he'd created

groaned and nearly came right up off the bed

groaned as he moved across her body

head dipped toward her breast

hands clenching in her buttocks now, he lifted her, felt slender legs grip his hips

he bit back a groan as she (*arched/bucked*) beneath him

he caught her clit, drawing it gently between his lips to suckle her

he could smell her (*arousal/excitement*)

he cupped a hand beneath her bottom, tilted her hips and began a slow rhythm

he'd barely gotten into her before her hot tunnel began clutching and gripping him

he dragged his tongue back to feather it over her quivering clit

he enjoyed watching a woman ride him

he fingered her curls and toyed with the wet heat he found

he found the hot, wet heat of her and slipped two fingers inside

he grazed his teeth across her bud and pushed a finger inside her at the same time

he groaned as she worked her entrance over the tip of his shaft

he groaned roughly as he slid in to the hilt

he knelt behind her, skin to skin, poised to mate

he lay on his back, watching her as her hands explored him at length

he loved the flare of her hips with the soft belly in between

held her tightly while his fingertips (*goaded/teased*) her to new heights of rapture held his breath as his groin jerked in greedy expectation

held his breath as she slowly fingered him from hilt to tip

he licked her clit, teasing it with his tongue and then (*flicked/sucked*) it

he pressed his mouth against her (*mound*)

her raspy breaths and strained cries drove him harder

he slipped a finger inside her panties, focused on her tight bundle of nerves

he stroked his tongue in and out, pushing her closer to the edge

her sweet sheened body arched, (*offering/begging*) him for more

her brows were drawn together in curiosity as she examined his body

her gasp slid along his senses as she braced herself against his chest

her heart pounded against his

her hips rocked as he touched her

her hunger and need meet and match his own

her long nails scratched across his back

her lithe body moved in a creative combination of (*back and forth/circular*) motions

her loss of control was unbelievable, unexpected

her sharp little teeth (*scored/grazed/nipped*) at his shoulder as he began to thrust inside her

her tongue trailed slowly down his body from his nipple to the apex of his thighs

he toyed with her, biding his time until he could fill her completely

he trembled as she worked her way from his neck to his abdomen and then down to the waste band of his jean he wanted to bury himself inside her as deeply as he could and not come out until he'd gotten his fill

he was helpless to resist her as she slid her hand into his jeans

his body ached with the need for release, for the ease he knew he could find in her

his body was on fire—hot, hard and ready

his climax boiled in his balls, tingled at the base of his spine

his finger moved within her damp folds and she whimpered

his fingers slicked across one small, sensitive piece of flesh at the core of her

his fingers stroking her in time with his thrusts

his gut ablaze with need, he latched tight to his control

his gut clenched tight, his reserve of willpower quickly dwindling

his groin jerked in greedy expectation

his hand slid up her leg, all the way to her wet cleft

his hands lifted her butt, his thumbs spread her folds, and his mouth captured her

his hand stroked her back, finding the deep curve that gave rise to her firm, tight bottom

his hand swept down her body to the center of her

his own body stiffened while waves of pleasure poured through him

his sex was throbbing like a toothache

his thick ridge nudged against her clitoris with delicious friction

lifted her and she clasped her legs around his waist as he (*entered/impaled/pierced/thrust into*) her

lifted her hips into his hand and he gave her more

like pure white heat, he felt her tightening, convulsing, milking his flesh

lightly brushed his fingers over her sensitive sex

long, smooth length of her legs wrapped around his hips

maintained the slow rhythmic in and out motion of his finger

one finger, then two, he dipped into her (*damp/moist*) heat

one hand slid between her thighs and found her creamy, slick with her own need

pleasure washed over him when her damp, wicked mouth surrounded the head of his dick

pressed his face against her mound, inhaled her sweet scent

reached out and unsnapped the front clasp of her bra

running (*fingers/palms*) (*inside/up*) her thighs, he gently parted her legs and knelt between them

sensations assaulted him

she bucked against his mouth, and he closed his hands over her hips, holding her still

she climaxed hard against his (*mouth/fingers*)

she was pure energy in his arms

she was wrapped around him, her silky sex rubbing against his

shivered at the sensation of her lips on his flesh

slicked his thumbs back and forth, spreading her moisture

slid down his body as she continued to lick and taste every part of him

slid her hand inside his underwear to cup his warm, hard, silky flesh

slowly rocking her lower body against his

spurred by the frantic need that strained within him

stroke after sensuous stroke

taking all she had to offer and silently demanding that she give even more

the first tremors began inside, moving along his manhood, in tiny convulsive jerks

the hot, heady perfume of her feminine arousal filled his head

the most primitive instinct known to man

the only way he would truly find ease was in the soft, hot clasp of her body

the snug grip of her sex stroking him

the taste of her was salty sweet, slippery and delicious

there was passion inside her equal to his own

they were intimately joined from breast to thigh, with his legs caught between hers

this was about giving her a memory that would soothe her far into the future

tilted her hips to receive him

took his rock hard velvet like steel into her fingers and led him to her

touched her glistening pink flesh with his thumbs

ultra soft, pink flesh, swelling with excitement

the unique flavor of her flashed through him

used her own (*slick heat/dampness*) to stroke her

wherever their bodies were touching, he felt as if lightning cracked just beneath his skin

wet, sweet and wild with need she shuddered beneath him

with a flick of his tongue he tasted her desire

with unsteady hands he ripped the packet and covered himself

worked another finger inside her

Heroine

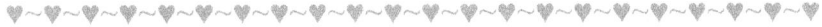

a bolt of fire lanced through her

a shiver of arousal shot through her at his dominant forcefulness

a shock of pleasure stole what breath remained in her lungs

a throb sprang up between her legs

a tiny moan caught in her throat

adjusting her curves to the hard, flat planes of his body

an unwanted moan escaped her throat

arched her body up to meet his

crisp hair trailed from his navel, to his groin framing his large sex

convulsed with pleasure from the stroke of his fingers

dazed in pleasure, her world narrowed to nothing but his touch

demanded that she submit to him, give up that last bit of herself

dug her fingers into his hair (*wrapped her legs around him/ her legs encircled his waist*)

dug her nails into his shoulders, arching hungrily up to meet his next thrust

eased her body closer to his

erotic bump and grind that was as old as mankind itself

everywhere he touched her, it felt as if an electrical current pulsed beneath her skin

felt a hot fire in her loins and contractions in her womb

felt a sting at her throat just as his fingertips found the center of her desire

felt her climax building and sensed his passion rising to its peak in unison with hers

felt his erection pressing between her legs

finally, she could hear, see, smell, taste and feel him within her fire such as she'd never imagined seared her feminine center

gasped when she felt his bare, hot skin under her palm

gentled her hold, stroking him carefully from base to tip

gently closed her hand around his shaft

glimpsed the startling proof of his desire

hammered at her will, forcing her to yield

hand closed around his erection, circling him, tracing each vein, grasping his testicles

heated licks of fiery sensation tormented her

heat flooded her insides, liquid fire pooled low in her belly

he gasped aloud as she took him in

he stripped out of his own clothes and stretched out along side her

he was thick, with velvety soft covering

heard a ragged murmur of satisfaction in his throat

heart slammed erratically in anticipation

heat consumed her, she was wet and ready

heat swept across her body

her bare breast tingled

her body arched, her thighs opened almost of their own volition

her body bombarded by sensation after sensation

her body, eager, desperate to know his touch, his possession

her body flamed, the heat moving from her thighs, up her abdomen to her breasts

her body milked him as small spasms ran through her

her body surged with (*throbbing/warm moist*) heat

her (*body swelled/pleasure doubled*) at the drugging scent of him

her fingers could barely circle him

her fingers raked through his thick, soft hair as her touch inflamed him

her hands slid off his damp skin

her heels dug into the small of his back as she lifted into him

her over-aroused crotch rubbed against the length of his penis

her raging hormones warm, tantalizing tongue

he was long, thick and solid, with velvety soft covering

his body shockingly hot over hers

his bulging sex, hidden from her eyes by a tiny scrap of g-string

his fingers (*found/toyed*) with the nub of her passion as his steel drove into her

his fingers found the bare flesh of her saturated sex

his practiced fingers moved quickly and before she knew it she was naked

his taste was hot and male

incredible sensations raced through her with a force that left her gasping for breath

lowering herself slowly, accepting the thick fullness of him

made a growling sound in the back of his throat as with one thrust he sheathed himself

male member heavy and erect

moaned at the taste of him as she took him into her mouth

pleasure tore her apart as the orgasm seemed never ending

pressed her groin against the thickness of his erection

seemed that her very essence centered on the feel of his body against hers

sensation and emotion wrapped around her

she arched bearing down on the fingers filling her

she (*arched/arching shamelessly*) into his hand

she clung to him, sinking into his body

Rebecca Andrews

she cried out, her body trembling as the pleasure rose inside her

she'd been close to orgasming, just from his mouth on her breast

she felt a spasmodic tightening of his muscles

she pulled back, let him watch her tongue curl around one side of the wide crest

she sank down on him, taking him slow and deep

she spiraled up and over carrying him with her

she strained against (*his hand/him*)

she took his hand and guided it

she whimpered, as he pierced her to the hilt

she whimpered into his mouth, hungry to feel his hands all over her bare body

she'd never experienced such intense chemistry before

sighed as his lips moved over her

sighed when he cupped her hips

slid her thumb over the head to test the slippery secretion there

slid the palms of her hands up his chest

slow throb pulsing through her body

squeezed gently and watched a drop of fluid appear on the tip

stroked between her legs, probing for the (*bud/swollen clit*) that throbbed with need

taking all he was giving, absorbing the heat of him

tantalized her with his tongue until she thought she'd die

the broad hot head of his erection prodded her slick, swollen folds

the dark hair of his chest made a very distracting trail down his abdomen

the exquisite knot of desire in her belly tightened

Lovemaking

the head of his cock bathed in her wet heat

the light in his eyes grew suddenly wild

the musk and sweat of his body filled her nostrils

the rough hair on his legs scraped the inside of her thighs as he nudged her legs wider

the sensation of his damp, slick skin sliding over hers

the steely bar of his erection jammed against her stomach

three hard, furious thrusts of his hips, pleasure splintered inside her

thrill after thrill shot though her as he possessed her body

watched the pleasure on his face as she toyed with his (*member/penis/cock*)

when he closed a hand over her breasts, heat shot straight down to her belly and lower

wild hunger flared through (*him/her*)

Finish

♥~♥~♥~♥~♥~♥~♥~♥~♥~♥~♥~♥~♥~♥~♥~♥~♥~♥~♥~♥

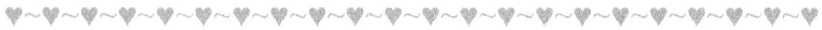

clamp(*ing*)	clasp	clench(*ing*)
clutch(*ing*)	compress	convulsed
consume	contraction(*s*)	grasp(*ing*)
gripp(*ing*)	milking	pulsing
quench	quake	quiver
release	rippling	riding
seize(*d*)	shiver	shudder(*ed*)
spasm	sucked	squeezing
throbbed	tighten(*ing*)	tremble
twinge	unfurl	

and then he tensed	felt her inhale then sigh
last vestiges of his control	no thoughts of control
relief and pleasure combined	shaking violently
slid deep inside	so far gone
steady build of her need	swelling within her
unexpected tightness	

brilliant pinpoints of light clashed and exploded behind her closed eyelids as she began to orgasm

clung to him desperately

couldn't stop the long, ragged groan of release

electricity sizzled from his balls, up his spine and centered in his brain

hard body heaved, went rigid

he covered her, slipped inside

he entered her, buried so deeply

he pumped and thrust, rocking her hips

Lovemaking

he rolled with her, trapping her beneath his plunging hips

he was so deep inside it made her ache

his body quivered with strain

his climax boiled in his balls and tingled at the base of his spine

his renewed passion ignited hers whenever it began to fade

his voice guttural and strained with passion

immerse himself, (*deep/deeper*)

leaned his head back as he felt her body clutching his

looked so rough and tumble sexy that she wanted him all over again

lust was tearing through him, adrenaline spiking, and they were both coming

sensations curled through her like a tidal wave and pushed her into rapture

shaky with desire, he groaned

she'd had so many orgasms she'd lost count

she slid down to him soft, boneless, limp

she lay back incapable of any movement

she was like warm pliant clay, her body damp with perspiration, her arms limp on the pillow

shook from the exertion of his release

shuddered and cried out her name

shudders wracked his body

the explosion that detonated in her overtook her

the heady rush of blood to his groin

throwing his head back, he took her, plunging in

trailed kisses along the side of her neck before rolling off

tumbled over the last edge of pleasure

unable to wait another moment

After Glow

♥~♥

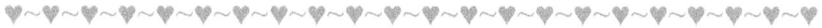

a generous lover, catering to every physical and emotional need

brushed aside the sweaty curls from his brow and kissed him gently, before laying her cheek on his shoulder

came to him readily this time, trusting without question

cherishing the steady beat of (*his/her*) heart beneath (*his/her*) ear

closed his eyes at how she felt against his flesh, warm and soft against him

cupped (*his/her*) cheek in (*his/her*) palm

dropped soft kisses on (*his/her*) face and throat

eyes felt heavy and (*he/she*) let them slide closed as (*he/she*) snuggled against (*him/her*)

feeling warm and more content than (*he/she*) could ever remember

felt small and vulnerable and soft in his arms

fit perfectly in his arms

(*he/she*) lay next to (*him/her*), the sheet pulled to their waists

he loved the feel of his fingers tangling in those rich, luxurious (*color*) strands

he paused to admire her laying there warm and soft nestled into the bedding

he tried to slip out from underneath her without waking her up

he'd awakened the hidden pleasures of her body

(*he'd/she'd*) never been more content

heartbeat strong and steady under (*his/her*) ear

held her close, reveling in the feel of her as he cradled her with his body

held her tight against him, as his heart continued to race

his big body curved protectively, commandingly, around her

his body still, tight with need, his blood still simmering

it was all she could do not to burrow her nose against his neck and just inhale him

looked up at her as he laughed from his exhaustion

picked her up with great gentleness, cradled her body close to his

pressed a kiss against the pulse in (*his/her*) neck

pressed (*his/her*) lips to (*his/hers*) sweetly

pulling her to him so she lay tucked against his side

ran her hands over his damp skin

settling her head on his shoulder

she could feel he was aroused again

she could feel his heartbeat and every breath he took

she opened her eyes and smiled up at him

she shifted in his arms and he saw the future so clearly

she'd forgotten passion could feel like this

she'd rocked his world

smoothed her hair between his fingers as she slept

swamped with emotions, she turned her face into his shoulder

the tenderness shattered them both

the warm imprint of (*his/her*) lips lingered on (*his/her*) skin

there was a good chance that with all their heat, they would be making a baby tonight

warm sweet emotion went through (*him/her*)

was already hard for her wanting to taste her again

was curved beside (*him/her*)

with a soft sigh she curled on her side and snuggled into the sheets

woke up in the morning wrapped up in warm, naked woman

Battle Skills

♥~♥

a thin trickle of blood ran from the corner of (*his/her*) lip

a vastly more skilled fighter

a wink of metal flashed in (*his/her*) palm

adjusted (*his/her*) headset, pulling the lip microphone closer to (*his/her*) mouth

aimed carefully and then lowered (*his/her*) gun

a rush of adrenaline shot through (*him/her*)

air wheezed out between (*his/her*) teeth

bared his teeth, snarled

bleeding, he kicked one attacker back to confront the newcomer

blood sprayed through the air in a fine crimson mist

breath hot as fire raced out of (*his/her*) lungs

brought her heel down on his instep

bullet slammed into (*him/her*), ripping flesh, tearing muscle

buried (*his/her*) fist in (*his/her*) stomach

came at (*him/her*) with ham-sized fists

cold steel pressed against (*his/her*) throat

coming up with a hard fist to the guy's solar plexus

cringed at the ragged wound the knife had left behind

crouched by the open doorway, a grenade launcher in (*his/her*) arms

danced back lightly on the balls of (*his/her*) feet

dodged the fist before it slammed into (*his/her*) (*eye/jaw/face*) drove the knife in twice, once in each (*lung/rib*) with a twist

eased the knife out and a gush of blood flowed over (*his/her*) fingers

easily ducked the wild blow

face was red, eyes slits of rage

fell backward from the impact

felt the satisfying crack of knuckles against bone

gave (*him/her*) a quick karate chop to the back of the neck

glancing shot to the temple

grabbed a handful of hair and flung her across the room

grabbed him by the throat and lifted him off his feet

hand flexed into a fist

(*he/she*) hadn't started this fight, but (*he/she*) was damned well going to finish it

head-butted the man and knocked him away

head hanging down, blood dripping from (*his/her*) split lip

heard the roar of the crowd behind (*him/her*)

(*he/she*) dodged, spun and with a well placed kick, dropped (*his/her*) attacker

(*he/she*) wielded the sword with the skill of an expert

his message was clear, he wasn't going to start this fight

(*his/her*) opponent would most certainly underestimate (*him/her*), but (*he/she*) wasn't about to make the same mistake

kick to the groin, and a whack across his back

kicked, driving the bones of his nose into his brain

kicked the weight-bearing leg out from under him

leaped forward, swinging viciously with (*his/her*) right arm

leveled the gun and squeezed off two rounds in a double tap

lowered his right shoulder and charged

managed to twist away and wrench free

methodically pumping a fist into his face

never good to go into a fight with the opponent sure you wouldn't kill him

planted a hand in the middle of the man's back and gave him a solid shove

pushed the man away with all (*his/her*) strength

ran (*his/her*) tongue over the inside of (*his/her*) stinging cheek

red faced, eyes slits of rage

screams and shouts erupted in the bar

senses went on heightened alert

sent his blade hurling

slammed (*him/her*) up against the wall

slammed into the far wall, fell to the floor and lay there, limp and unmoving

slamming his fist into his sternum with a series of powerful blows

slipped the dagger from (*his/her*) (*belt/sheath/pocket*)

snarled and charged again

spun slowly on the balls of (*his/her*) feet

stars exploding in front of (*his/her*) eyes

steel caressed the vulnerable place where (*his/her*) pulse beat

struggled to stand, but (*his/her*) legs wouldn't cooperate

swiped at *(his/her)* ribs with a lethal looking knife

the blade buried deep in (*his/her*) abdomen

the blow was teeth jarring

the first blow shattered (*his/her*) kneecap

the front of (*his/her*) (*shirt/blouse*) turning red, quickly

the look in his eyes said he didn't just want to bloody him; he wanted to kill him the set of his meaty shoulders was distinctly aggressive

the shock ran up his arm, ending with a riff of satisfaction

the thug held the knife reversed, the blade laying along his forearm, the tip pointing toward his elbow

there was going to be no way around dropping the guy by force

the underlying tension of a (*soldier/warrior*)

took the first blow in the gut

twisted open a butterfly knife and plunged it into (*his/her*) side

unbuttoned (*his/her*) (*shirt/blouse*) and applied pressure to the wound

waited until all of (*his/her*) weight was on (*his/her*) left foot, then swept (*his/her*) right leg forward

with a vicious blow to his nose he felt the bone give way with a grinding sensation beneath his knuckles

with the back of (*his/her*) hand (*he/she*) wiped the blood from (*his/ her*) mouth

wrapped an arm around his neck and drew him up right

Other Worldly

Psychic Abilities & Definitions
♥~♥~♥~♥~♥~♥~♥~♥~♥~♥~♥~♥~♥~♥~♥~♥~♥~♥~♥~♥

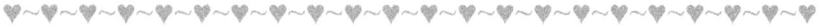

Adept: the general word used to label an functional psychic; the specific ability is much more specialized.

Astral Projection or Mental Projection: An out-of-body experience in which an "**astral body**" becomes separate from the physical body.

Automatic Writing: Writing produced without conscious thought.

Aura Reading: Perception of the energy fields surrounding people, places, and things.

Clairvoyance/Second Sight: the ability to know things, to pick up bits of information, seemingly out of thin air.

Death Warning: A vision of a living person prior to their death.

Divination: Gaining insight into a situation via a ritual.

Dowsing: Ability to locate objects.

Dream Projecting: the ability to enter another's dream.

Dream Walking: the ability to invite/draw others into ones own dreams.

Empathy: an empath experiences the emotions of others.

Energy Medicine: Healing by channeling a form of energy

Healing: the ability to heal injuries to self or others: often but not always ancillary to mediumistic abilities.

Healing Empathy: an empath/healer has the ability to not only feel but also to heal the pain/injury of another.

Latent: the term used to describe unwakened or inactive abilities, as well as to describe a psychic not yet aware of being psychic.

Medium or Channeling: A medium has the ability to communicate with the dead.

Precognition: A seer or precog has the ability to correctly predict future events.

Psycho Kinesis or **Telekinesis:** Manipulation of matter or energy by the power of the mind.

Psychometric: the ability to pick up impressions from objects.

Regenerative: the ability to heal ones own injuries/sickness (a classification unique and separate from a healers abilities)

Remote Viewing: Gathering of information at a distance.

Recognition: Perception of past events.

Scrying: Use of an item to view events at a distance or in the future.

Telepathy: Transfer of thoughts or emotions.

Transvection: Bodily levitation or flying.

Spider Sense: the ability to enhance one's normal senses (*sight, hearing, smell*) through concentration and the focusing of ones own mental and physical energy.

Telekinesis: the ability to move objects with the mind.

Telepathic Mind Control: the ability to influence/control others through mental focus and effort. Extremely rare ability.

Telepathy: (touch and non touch) the ability to pick up thoughts from others. Some telepaths only receive, while others have the ability to send thoughts.

Psychic Descriptions
♥~♥~♥~♥~♥~♥~♥~♥~♥~♥~♥~♥~♥~♥~♥~♥~♥~♥~♥~♥

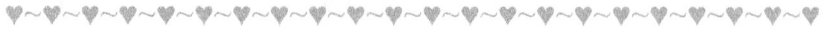

a flood of hot, rough sensations slid down (*his/her*) spine

another sharp image sizzled through (*his/her*) brain

a sudden sensation, a chill that crawled slowly over her body

a warm, familiar energy coursed up (*his/her*) arm

aura coated in (*twisting/greasy*) black flames

cocooning (*him/her*) in a telepathic (*bubble/sense*) of safety

darkness folded over her, a quiet restfulness

felt that same premonition of fear of danger

gasping softly in the dark as her thoughts folded around him

(*he'd/she'd*) never known an aura of energy like (*his/hers*) before

(*he/she*) held (*him/her*) mentally

he pushed his mind, willed himself deeper into hers

he touched her mind with his, just a feathery stroke meant to comfort

her gift came to her genetically as part of her heritage

her mind took him inside as if he belonged there

her prickly defenses going up immediately

her 6th sense warned her of the approaching evil

(*his/her*) calling one of healing

(*his/her*) head tilted to one side as if (*he/she*) were listening to distant voices

(*his/her*) intuition worked to protect (*him/her*) and keep (*him/her*) safe

(*his/her*) mind sank into a light trance

(*his/her*) unconscious mind greedily clasped (*his/hers*)

impenetrable darkness of her aura swirled once, brushed against him

never used second sight like this before

power spiked, scraping across (*his/her*) shields and (*skin/flesh*)

raised the hair on the nape of (*his/her*) neck

relaxed and let (*his/her*) precognitive talent work

reluctant to delve deeper into (*his/her*) mind than (*he/she*) already had

sensation tingled over (*his/her*) skin, a wash of fever-heat

spine tingling rush of power coated (*his/her*) entire body

the link between them resonated with pain

the vision trembled just outside (*his/her*) mental grasp

was strong enough to take control of (*his/her*) mind

Angels

♥~♥~♥~♥~♥~♥~♥~♥~♥~♥~♥~♥~♥~♥~♥~♥~♥~♥~♥

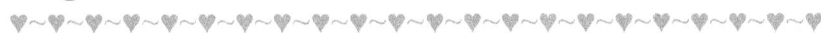

angels of light	archangels	beautiful
blessed realm	chamber	cherub
eternity	faithful	flaming
glittering gates	guardian angels	holy knight
sacrifice	shining shield	sword
warrior/warrior angels		

anti–chamber to heaven	frail and fragile creatures
head bowed in silence	heavenly messengers
supreme commander	twilight world of purgatory
vows of loyalty and courage	

beauty and peace of the blessed realm

every feather in (*his/her*) wings in place

(*he'd/she'd*) died with (*his/her*) faith in God unshaken

helping to fight the eternal battle against...

(*his/her*) robes were immaculate

left the battle field to answer the summons
promise of freedom and power and glory
repent (*his/her*) sins and gain admittance to heaven

Vampires

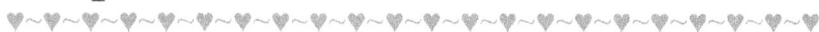

air thickened
drink blood to survive
hungered to touch her
night enfolded him
strong command to feed
tuned his acute hearing

billowing out
glided toward her
inhuman speed
self-imposed penance
tall, gaunt

a growl vibrated up (*his/her*) throat and (*his/her*) fangs flashed

a kill would draw (*his/her*) victims' nightmares into (*his/her*) soul

a known feeder who prayed on human blood

a shadow grew over the room

a supernaturally charged force field protected (*him/her*)

allowing (*his/her*) senses to flare out

at the setting of the sun, humans were the prey

blood had been spilled, the air thick with the scent

bounties had been placed on them and they had been hunted ruthlessly

could feel (*his/her*) hunger, (*his/her*) inner need to touch (*him/her*)

could (*feel/hear*) the blood (*roaring/rushing*) in (*his/her*) veins

could show (*him/her*) pleasure like (*he'd/she'd*) never known

could tell by the heightened color of (*his/her*) skin that (*he'd/she'd*) fed not long ago

darkness called to (*him/her*), summoned (*him/her*) home to the alleys and gutters where (*his/her*) kind belonged

decided she must have imagined his presence in her mind

drawing his tongue across his fingertips, he smeared his saliva over the double puncture wounds

every cell in (*his/her*) body demanded nourishment

eyes glowed the fiery red of a predator on the hunt

felt (*his/her*) incisors lengthen in hunger

fire, sunlight and beheading could destroy them

flew across the sky with silent stealth

for an instant the fading daylight sparked a glint of crimson in (*his/her*) eyes

found (*himself/herself*) wondering what synthetic blood tasted like

glowing eyes, eerie and haunting

golden glow of (*his/her*) immortal soul

had encountered vampires before, but never one this old or this powerful

(*he/she*) could change shape, travel faster than the human eye could follow

(*he/she*) felt it now, evil spreading like a force across the air

(*he/she*) ghosted along dark streets, (*his/her*) senses alert

(*he/she*) tore a wound in (*his/her*) wrist and pressed it to (*his/her*) mouth

(*he/she*) was a vampire and strictly off limits

(*he/she*) was fading away, (*his/her*) life force simply waning

heart raced with anxiety, a sound (*he/she*) knew (*he/she*) could hear

his bare chest was pale rather than tan

(*his/her*) blood warmed instantly and coiled into an ache low in (*his/her*) abdomen (*his/her*) body cried out for blood, for nourishment

(*his/her*) head fell back, exposing (*his/her*) throat to (*his/her*) tongue

(*his/her*) nostrils flared, savoring the salty tang of (*his/her*) flesh

hot crimson scent of blood

hunger roared through (*him/her*)

hunger that burned within (*him/her*), rousing at the tantalizing scent of prey

knew (*he/she*) shouldn't have shape-shifted until full dark

learned a lot about (*men/women*) in (*his/her*) many lifetimes

let (*his/her*) body melt into its wingless, fully human shape

let out the snarl of a wild beast

lips brushed against the delicate skin of her inner wrist

lips drew back in a silent snarl

lips feasted from (*his/her*) wrist

mouth broke from her skin, his warm breath cooling the wetness

never felt such an overwhelming imperative to mate

night wind swirled around the figure

no ordinary hunger, but one of (*gut-wrenching/skin-crawling*) necessity

notoriously charming and seductive

only the old ones possessed an eerie stillness

random heat traces (*he/she*) identified as small animals

rather than painful, the bite had been wonderfully erotic

ruby red liquid shimmering in the crystal goblet

she looked up at the sun and shielded her eyes to its power

shrouding (*himself/herself*) in a psychic veil

silver and holy water burned their skin like acid

soft creamy skin, veins pulsing blue beneath it

spent most of (*his/her*) time studying, trying to find a way to reverse the magic that cursed (*him/her*) and all like (*him/her*)

stringy hair and long fingernails

strong enough to take control of (*his/her*) mind

supernatural power radiated from (*him/her*) like heat from a furnace

swept (*his/her*) tongue across the pinpricks at (*his/her*) throat to close the wound with (*his/her*) healing saliva

swept through the dark sky like a wraith

the last traces of (*his/her*) blood slithered down (*his/her*) throat

the sun had barely set, the afterglow making (*his/her*) head ache and (*his/her*) eyes sting

the sweetness of her natural fragrance confirmed her robust health

the thought of him biting her neck while thrusting slow and deep made her hot

their thoughts flowed together

through the darkness (*he/she*) could sense (*him/her*), feel (*him/her*) moving among the shadows

tore a wound in (*his/her*) wrist and pressed it to (*his/her*) mouth

to talk telepathically to (*him/her*)

veiled from (*his/her*) sight, (*he/she*) stood at the foot of (*his/her*) bed

was a different world after dark, one feared by mortals

with a gasp she arched her neck inviting him to graze there

wrapped the night around (*his/her*) body and disappeared

Other

♥~♥

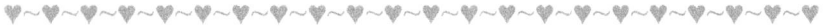

a hazy form	apparition	archfiends
ascend	authority	command
control	dark angels	demonic form
divination	dominance	dream
extraordinary	flow	forces of darkness
forsaken	forecast	foresight
foretelling	glide	hallucination
insight	lavish	lush
luxurious	opulent	plush
prophecy	power	rare
revelation	rich	rule
something drifted	suffering	torture
unusual	visualization	waft

a familiar, unwelcoming burning sensation signaled the onset of the change

a glittering trail of silver sparkles sifted from the agitated pixy

a mark of power (*he/she*) recognized immediately

acute sense of smell

blood of gypsies flowing thick through (*his/her*) veins

bloody muzzle and glowing eyes

body felt as if it had jelled to ice

called upon the beast that dwelled within (*him/her*)

cleansing influence of the slow-burning flame

concentrated on the light dancing on the narrow wick

dark, ancient oak wood carved with symbols

ears pinned, hackles raised, lips curled back to show their teeth

fingers curled and hardened, sharpened into talons

flicked (*his/her*) wrist, bringing the sphere back to rest in (*his/her*) palm

heir to an unbroken chain of masters

(*his/her*) heightened senses felt (*him/her*) all the way through (*his/her*) entire body

(*his/her*) jaw splintered, lengthened

(*his/her*) sworn enemy

howled with pain as (*his/her*) bones stretched and shifted and the werewolf took control of (*his/her*) body

impressive tribal tattoo that covered the entire left side of his torso

invisible stroke of fingers against (*his/her*) (*face/jaw/cheek*)

lifted his (*nose/beak*) to the wind

little more than a shadowy figure in the moonlight

long, rich robes draped his stocky frame

new found human abilities

paws, the size of his hands

pendant (*he/she*) wore caught the moonlight and glinted

power of the moonlight shimmering through (*his/her*) veins

power swirled and danced around (*him/her*)

pull of the moon was a heat that would only get worse in the coming nights

skin changed to hide and fur

sprang forward, (*his/her*) body shifting from (*man/woman*) to (*wolf/animal*) form in midair

temperature in the room had dropped twenty degrees

the awakening of the beast inside (*him/her*) was magical, not subject to the laws of physics

the (*cane/staff/wand*) in his hand hummed with delicate power

the cold wrapped around (*him/her*)

the crone morphed into a middle-aged woman

the fairy fluttered down on wings like a moth

the minions of death lived for the opportunity to kill

the shimmering veil solidified

the throne room a white marble cavern with moving mosaics on the walls

the usual red sheen of energy shifted gold

the very air around the (*man/woman*) seemed charged with mystical energy

the warding on the shop was complex and unique

the werewolf's lips drew back in a predatory grin

there'd been no warning from the cards, runes or any other divination

throats, claws and fangs slashing and ripping

trusted warrior's staff

was forever asking (*him/her*) to ferret out traitors and information

waved a hand and a ball of white whipped out and blinded (*him/her*)

with a delicate wave, (*he/she*) flashed away

with a growl, the wolf shook himself free

with a victorious howl, it buried its fangs in the other wolf's (*neck/shoulder*)

with (*his/her*) powers waning from the pain of (*his/her*) injuries

Imagery

Clouds, Storms

♥~♥~♥~♥~♥~♥~♥~♥~♥~♥~♥~♥~♥~♥~♥~♥~♥~♥~♥

breeze	clouds (*black, dark, green, purple*)	
cyclone	downpour	fog~ thick, dense
gale	gentle	gust
hail	haze	howling wind
hurricane	mild	mist
monsoon	murkiness	overcast
ozone	pleasant	rainstorm
rolling clouds	smog	soft
squall	strong wind	swirling mists
tempest	thick bank of fog	thunderstorm
tornado	tropical storm	twister
typhoon	vapor	whirlwind
wild winds		

Wet

♥~♥~♥~♥~♥~♥~♥~♥~♥~♥~♥~♥~♥~♥~♥~♥~♥~♥~♥

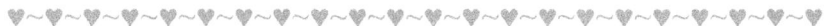

clammy	cloudburst	damp
deluge	drenched	dripping
heavy shower	humid	moist
saturated	shower	soaked/soaking
soaked to the skin	sodden	soggy
sopping	tacky	torrent

waterlogged	watery	wet
wringing wet		

Cold

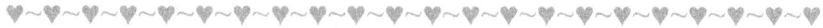

arctic	bitter	blizzard
bracing	chilly	freezing
frigid	frosty	frozen
glacial	ice-cold	icy
nippy	nor'easter	polar
snowstorm	sub-zero	wintry

Hot, Dry

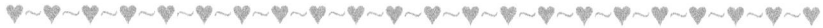

baking	blazing	blistering
broiling	burning-up	heat
intense	roasting	scalding
scorched	searing	sizzling
sweltering	torrid	

Day

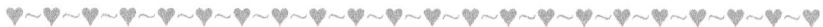

crack of dawn	dawn	daybreak
daylight	energy	glare
light of day	morning	sunbeams
sunrise	sunshine	sunup
twilight	waves	

Night

♥~♥

darkness	dusk	end of day
evening	gloom	nightfall
nighttime	shade	shadows
sundown	sunset	

Scenery

♥~♥

ambiance	countryside	earth
geography	ground	landscape
location	nature	panorama
place	scenery	site
soil	spot	surroundings
terrain	vista	wildlife
world		

Landscape Descriptions

♥~♥

a dark smudge of clouds

a dazzling panorama of stars

a fork of lightening split the sky directly in front of her

a full moon shone and stars twinkled in the velvety sky

a lacy overlay of gray-tinged clouds

an enormous boom of thunder, accompanied by a flash of lightening

an owl hooted

a pale crescent moon slipped in and out of view

a pretty night, a little chill, a little breezy

a shooting star streaked across the black velvet sky overhead

a thin spring drizzle fell

afternoon storm beginning to gather on the horizon

berries ripened on thorny brambles

blowing snow was a blinding white swirl across the frozen expanse of...

blue sky stretched as far as the eye could see

clouds scudded in front of a quarter moon

cold air whistled into the house

dark nights lit only by limitless stars

first drops of rain dotted the pavement

flashing whitecaps caught what little moonlight filtered through a thin layer of clouds

froth churned on the water's surface

full moon flooded the valley with silver light

gazed through the rain slicked windshield

glittering stars peeked through the dense canopy of leaves

golden beams of (*sunlight/moonlight*) hit the panes of stained glass.

grass covering the foothills was turning green

hot with the thick damp heat that always lay like a blanket over (*place*)

huddled miserably in the wind

intense silver glow of the full moon

lake water slapped against the rocks

large oak trees shaded the house

lashing wind, driving rain, explosions of lightning

last rays of the sunset faded to a deep navy blue

late summer breeze ruffled the leaves

life moved slow and calm

moon rode toward fullness

moonlight painted a shimmering stripe across the surface of the lake

moonlight streamed through the bedroom window, hitting the bed

mosquitoes dive-bombed, oblivious to the heavy coating of insect repellant

night pressed hard against the last rays of daylight

night sky cloaked with clouds

night wind (*ruffled/lashed*) at her

not cold enough for frost, but the hillside was covered with dew

ocean was restless, waves pounded the shore

picked their way carefully across the snow covered parking lot

pinpricks of stars and a wan sickle moon drifting against the darkened sky

pools of streetlight shivering on the wet pavement

rain falling in sheets and rising fast

red orange rays of the setting sun (*fell across/crowned*) the hilltops

rhythmic rise and fall of waves rippling toward shore

sea thundering and spraying water into the air

silver and blue peaks of the mountains

silvery light pierced the thick cover of darkness

sky broke without warning

sky was diamond clear

smell of approaching rain

snowcapped peaks of the mountains soared into the clear blue sky line

snowflakes as big as cotton balls

soft pretty snowflakes dotting her windshield

spring thunder exploded overhead

stars twinkled above the city lights

steaming heat enclosed them in damp discomfort

sudden ear-shattering explosion of thunder

sun shining in through the scratched windows of his apartment

sunlight shimmered through falling snow

the air tasted so pure, so clean

the air was thick with smoke

the arctic storm had held (*whichever city*) in it's icy grip for days

the fire crept closer, across the floor

the heat was intense, flames (*soaring/rolling*) up ward

the (*howl/scream*) of the wind echoed around the house

the low hum of insects

the rattle of (*rain/hail*) on the windowpanes

the smell of hay and fresh manure filled his nostrils

the sun melted, spilling color over the western sky

the water was viciously, brutally cold

the wind struck him like a fist

when he'd first seen the moon it looked like a fiery ball

whipping wind and driving rain

wide open prairies stretched as far as the eye could see

winter sky hung heavy, spitting dime size snowflakes

wipers shoved wet, fat flakes off the glass

world was a carpet of color, gilded by the sun riding low in the west

Other

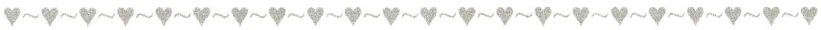

a century old farm house

a crystal chandelier hung low over a massive center table

a dim, smoke-choked bar

a featureless spot in the black ocean of jungle below

a loud blast and the shattering of glass

a quiet, tidy little town

a silver coffee service

a two story structure with wood trim and (*warm/cool*) painted walls

a wide balcony overlooked the cliff and the raging ocean below

air inside the chapel was thick with portents, and a goodly amount of dust

an airy sunroom located at the rear of the house

an antler hat rack

an old two-story frame house with a wide front porch

an open veranda stretching the width of the house

bed had (*any color*) satin sheets, a dark (*any color*) silk comforter

bed was made of stripped pine logs

brought the helicopter smoothly to hover

bunkhouse with faded logs and wide front porch

car somersaulted off the road, rolling over and over

cowhide and burled wood chair

cowhide rug lay on the floor

deep, cushy leather furniture

farm set in a deep, lush little valley

fire burning softly at her back

fire truck and police cars, with lights (*flashing/strobing*) in the distance

flames crackling in a rough stone fireplace

floor to ceiling stone fireplace

four towering columns rose skyward

framed family photographs and fussy throw pillows

furnishings were sleek and comfortable

gardens with meticulous tended blooms

gleaming wood floors polished to a high shine

groomed lawn that rose in tiered layers

grounds were surrounded by a high fence, topped with razor wire

hardwood floors and overstuffed leather furniture

hung his snow dusted coat in the closet

iron bed, modern dresser and a television

lovely old stoneware pots

lunchtime traffic was heavy

mansion's white stucco walls gleamed in the moonlight

modern high-rise condos enclosed the park

monstrosity of a house mounted on the crest of a hill

mossy, whitewashed brick, twin gables and a steeply pitched roof

oak floors shone beneath an impressive chandelier

obviously had an expensive barber and a more expensive tailor

old men at the counter talking baseball

one-hundred square mile ranch

parked in front of the diner, a longstanding gathering place

pulled his car to the curb and slammed on the brakes

ranch seemed to go on for miles, acre after acre

row after row of boats resting on the blue water of the marina

seagulls shrieked overhead

second floor sun-porch overlooked a circular driveway

shutters closed off the windows against the winter winds

stifling, crummy two-bedroom apartment

stomped her boots on the mat so she wouldn't track snow all over

the bar was smoky and dark

the phone jarred him awake

the sacredness and beauty of life was all around her

the stone walls of the secret underground chamber were cold and dank

the walls were covered in softly striped wallpaper

thirty-foot ceiling framed by log beams

walls covered in softly striped wallpaper

white sheers fluttered in the (*cold/warm*) breeze

Rebecca Andrews

Clothing

General

anorak, belt, blouse, cardigan, dress, gloves, jacket, jeans, jumper, overalls, overcoat, pullover, raincoat, scarf, shirt, shorts, skirt/miniskirt, socks, suit, sweater, sweatshirt, T-shirt, tie, trousers

Dresses and Skirts

baby doll, backless, bare-backed, burlap bag, caftan, cardigan, chemise, cocktail dress, cotton dress, crinoline, crisp business suit, denim-mini, empire dress, evening gown, floral print skirt, halter dress, jumper, kimono, knit dress, lace dress, long sheath, maternity dress, maxi, micro-mini, midi, mini-dress, muu muu, pleated silk crepe, potato sack, sequined-mini, sheath, shift, sheer wrap, shirt dress, slip-dress, slit-dress

246

strapless dress	stretch mini	sundress
sweater-dress	T-shirt dress	tent-dress
toga	tube-dress	turtleneck dress

black velvet evening gown	cinched with a wide belt
elegantly tailored dress	slitted, black leather mini
strapless lamé dress	

Pants and Shorts

♥~♥~♥~♥~♥~♥~♥~♥~♥~♥~♥~♥~♥~♥~♥~♥~♥~♥~♥~♥

bell bottoms	Bermuda shorts	buckskins
camouflage	capris	cargo
chaps	chinos	clam-diggers
cords	cutoffs	deck pants
drawstring pants	dungarees	fatigues
harem pants	hip huggers	jockey pants
levis	overalls	painters
pedal pushers	spandex	stirrup pants
stretch pants	surfers	

Shirts and Tops

♥~♥~♥~♥~♥~♥~♥~♥~♥~♥~♥~♥~♥~♥~♥~♥~♥~♥~♥~♥

blouse	bustier	camisole
camp shirt	chemise	clerical (*priest*)
cowboy	cut-off	dress shirt
flannel	formal	halter-top
Hawaiian	hunting shirt	jockey
midriff	polo-shirt	tank-top
tunic	turtleneck	western-dress shirt
wife-beater		

Sweaters

♥~♥

argyle	cardigan	cowl-neck
crew-neck	fisherman's	jacquard
shell	tennis	turtleneck

Undergarments and Nightwear

♥~♥

baby doll	bikini underwear	body-suit
boxer shorts	boy-shorts	BVDs
bustier	camisole	chemise
convertible bra	corset	crotchless panties
demi-cup bra	flannel pajamas	French-cut panties
garter	garter-belt	girdle
g-string	high-cut	hipsters
kimono	long johns	lounging pajamas
negligee	nightdress	nightgown
peek-a-boo bra	push-up bra	satin pajamas
satin robe	sleep shirt	slip
tanga (panties)	teddy	terrycloth robe
thong	T-shirt	thermal knit pajamas
thigh-highs		

Sportswear

♥~♥

bikini	jogging suit	swimming trunks
swimsuit	tracksuit	

Footwear

♥~♥

ankle boot	athletic shoe	ballet slipper
boat	boots	bootee
brogan	clunky heels	cleats
clodhoppers	clog	combat
cowboy	deck	dress
flats/skimmer	flip-flop	galoshes
go-go	half-boot	high-top
hip boot	hose	hosiery
loafer	Mary-Jane	moccasin
mule	open-toed	oxford
penny-loafer	platform	pump/high heel
saddle shoe	sandals	sling-back
slippers	sneakers	suede mules
socks	stiletto boots	stiletto heels
thigh-high boots	waders	wedgies
wingtips		

Descriptions

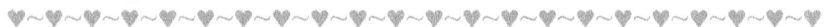

♥~♥

a beautiful young woman wearing a low-cut, aqua cocktail dress

a black silk robe

a brilliant (*color*) designer dress and high heels

a cashmere overcoat

a collarless suit in pale green

a crisp white tux shirt

discreet pearl drops at her ears

a dark-blue western suit

a sarong-style cover-up

a tailored Armani tuxedo

black, hooded sweatshirt that slipped off one shoulder to reveal her smooth, tanned skin

black tuxedo trousers with a satin stripe along the side

body hugging, black tank top

cream suit with a pale green shirt and a pair of sunglasses

crisply starched white shirt and subdued tie

dark wool-blended suit

form-fitting, tailored white suit that emphasized her hourglass figure

(*he/she*) never saw (*him/her*) in anything but jeans, a T-shirt and cowboy boots

he wore black, close-fitting clothing devoid of any military markings

jeans, running shoes, a T-shirt with a little blue flower print

khaki pants and a black polo

middle-aged woman wearing a form-fitting dress

rolled up T-shirt, revealing a stylized barbwire tattoo

she was wearing an uplift bra and a pair of control top briefs

she wore a flowered dress with a snappy little jacket

silk blouse with a white, cotton tank top beneath

silver bolo tie

slacks and a button-down shirt, with a leather overcoat and booted feet

sleeveless black T-shirt that accented the bulging muscles of his arms, black leather pants

stepped into the ivory cocktail dress, sliding her arms through spaghetti thin shoulder straps

the room was filled with big men wearing gleaming white, naval dress uniforms

two very small triangles stretched across her full breasts attached with a string that tied around her neck and back

Create Your Own Tags!!!

Colors

Black

anthracite	black as coal	black as jet
black as a crow	black as night	black as pitch
black as the ace of spades		blackish
blue-black	carbon	charcoal
coal	dingy	dusky
ebony	ink/inky	jet
licorice	midnight	obsidian
onyx	pearl	pitch
pitch-black	raven	sable
shadow	soot(*y*)	

Blue

azure	baby	blue-black
blueberry	blue-green	blueness
bluing	Caribbean blue	cerulean
cobalt	cornflower	dark
deep	delft	denim
dusty	electric	federal
French	indigo	lapis lazuli
light	livid	marine
midnight	mulberry	navy

neon	pale	Paris
peacock	periwinkle	powder
Prussian	robin's egg	royal
Sapphire	sky	slate
steel	teal	turquoise
ultramarine	Wedgwood	

Bronze

♥~♥

burnished	copper-colored	gold
reddish-brown	russet	rust

Brown

♥~♥

almond	auburn	bay
beige	brownish	brown-sugar
brick	bronze	brown-haired
brunette	buckskin	buff
burnt ochre	burnt orange	burnt russet
café au lait	Caledonia	cappuccino
chestnut	chocolate	cinnamon
cocoa	coffee	copper
dark	dark brown	dark-
complexioned	dark-haired	dark-skinned
deer hide	drab	dun
dusky	dust	earth
ecru	fawn	foxy
ginger	hazel	henna
khaki	Latin	leather

light brown
maple
mushroom
ochre
pigmented
raisin
russet
saddle
snuff-colored
taupe
toffee
walnut

liver-colored
Mediterranean
nut
olive-skinned
potato-skin
reddish-brown
rosewood
sepia
swarthy
tawny
tortoise-shell

mahogany
mocha
nutmeg
pecan
puce
roan
rust
sorrel
tan/tanned
terra-cotta
umber

Gray

ash
gunmetal
pearl
slate
tattletale

charcoal
hoary
pewter
smoke

dove
iron
silvery
sooty

Green

alfalfa
army
cabbage
celadon
cucumber
forest

apple
avocado
cactus
chartreuse
emerald
grass

aqua/aquamarine
bluish-green
celery
clover
fir
grasshopper

hunter	ivy	jade
John Deer	kelly	leaf
lime	malachite	mint
mist	moss	olive
pea	pear	peridot
pistachio	sage	sea
shamrock	teal	turquoise
verdant		

Orange

amber	apricot	bird of paradise
cantaloupe	carrot	cheese
copper	coral	peach
pumpkin	mango	nectarine
ocher	orange	salmon
sweet potato	tangerine	tiger
yam		

Purple

amaranthine	amethyst	aster
heliotrope	hydrangea	indigo
lavender	lilac	magenta
mauve	orchid	plum
tyrian	violet	wood

Red, Pink

♥~♥

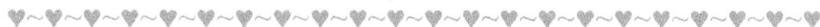

apple	ashes of roses	auburn
beet	blood	blush
brass	brick	bubble gum
burgundy	candy apple	cardinal
carmine	carnation	cayenne
cerise	cherry	cherry blossom
cherry tomato	cinnabar	claret
cochineal	cotton-candy	coral
cranberry	crimson	currant
dusky rose	fire-engine	garnet
hot pink	lobster	maroon
ox-blood	pepto bismol	raspberry
red amber	rhubarb	rose
rubescent	ruby	russet
rust	salmon	scarlet
shrimp	sunset	strawberry
terra cotta	titian	vermilion
watermelon	wine	

White, Off White

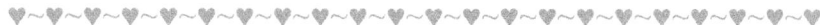

♥~♥

alabaster	albino	biscuit
bone	chalk	cream/creamy
coconut	colorless	cotton
daisy	dove	ecru
eggshell	fair	fair-skinned
frost	high in tone	ivory

light	light-complexioned	lily
lily-white	magnolia	marshmallow
milk/milky	milky quartz	moonstone
oatmeal	opal	oyster
pale	pallid	parchment
pearly	popcorn	sallow
salt	sugar	snow
swan	tattletale-gray	vanilla
washed-out	white jade	white-skinned
whitish		

Yellow, Gold

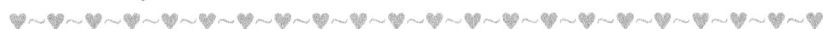

amber	ash blonde	banana
blanched	blonde	buff
bullion	butter	burnished
brass	cadmium	champagne
citrine	corn	cream
daffodil	faded	flaxen
fool's gold	honey	jonquil
lemon	mustard	ochre
palomino	primrose	pyrite
sandy	silver blonde	snowy
straw	sun-light	tawny
topaz	white-gold	

U.S. Military Ranks

Non-Commissioned Personnel

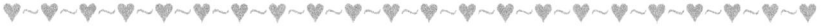

Service members E-1 through E-3 are usually in some kind of training status or on their initial assignment. The basic training phase is where recruits learn about military culture, its values and are taught skills required by their respective service branch.

Air Force

E-1	Airman Basic	AB
E-2	Airman	Amn
E-3	Airman First Class	A1C
E-4	Senior Airman	SrA

Army

E-1	Private	Pvt
E-2	Private	PV2
E-3	Private First Class	PFC
E-4	Corporal / Specialist	CPL / SPC

Marines

E-1	Private	Pvt
E-2	Private First Class	PFC
E-3	Lance Corporal	LCpl
E-4	Corporal	Cpl

Navy/Coast Guard

Coast Guard rank insignia are the same as the Navy except for color and the seaman recruit rank, which has one stripe.

E-1	Seaman Recruit	SR
E-2	Seaman Apprentice	SA
E-3	Seaman	SN
E-4	Petty Officer 3rd Class	PO3

Non-Commissioned Officers
E-5 thru E-7

Leadership and responsibility increases in the mid-level enlisted ranks. This responsibility is given formal recognition by use of the terms non-commissioned officer and petty officer. An Army sergeant, an Air Force staff sergeant, and a Marine corporal are considered NCO ranks. The Navy NCO equivalent, petty officer, is achieved at the rank of petty officer third class.

Air Force

E-5	Staff Sergeant	SSgt
E-6	Technical Sergeant	TSgt
E-7	Master Sergeant / First Sergeant	MSgt

Army

E-5	Sergeant	SGT
E-6	Staff Sergeant	SSG
E-7	Sergeant First Class	SFC

Marines

E-5	Sergeant	SGT
E-6	Staff Sergeant	SSgt
E-7	Gunnery Sergeant	GySgt

Navy/Coast Guard

E-5	Petty Officer 2nd Class	PO2
E-6	Petty Officer 1st Class	PO1
E-7	Chief Petty Officer	CPO

E-8

At the E-8 level, the Air Force, Army and Marines have two positions at the same pay grade. The senior master sergeant or a first sergeant in the Air Force depends on the person's job.

The same is true for the positions at the E-9 level. Marine Corps master gunnery sergeants and sergeants major receive the same pay but have different responsibilities. All told, E-8s and E-9s have 15 to 30 years on the job, and are commanders' senior advisers for enlisted matters.

Air Force

E-8

Senior Master Sergeant	SMSgt
First Sergeant	1SG

Army

E-8

Master Sergeant	MSG
First Sergeant	1SG

Marines

E-8

Master Sergeant	MSgt
First Sergeant	1Sgt

Navy/Coast Guard

E-8

Senior Chief Petty Officer	SCPO

E-9

A third E-9 is the senior enlisted person of each service. The sergeant major of the Army, the sergeant major of the Marine Corps, the master chief petty officer of the Navy and the chief master sergeant of the Air Force are at the highest levels of their services.

Air Force

Chief Master Sergeant	CmSgt
	First Sergeant
Command Chief Master Sergeant	CCM
Chief Master Sergeant of the Air Force	CMSAF

Army

Sergeant Major	SGM
Command Sergeant Major	CSM
Sergeant Major of the Army	SMA

Marines

Sergeant Major	SgtMaj
Master Gunnery Sergeant	MGySgt
Sergeant Major of the Marine Corps	SgtMajMC

Navy/Coast Guard

Master Chief Petty Officer	MCPO
Master Chief Petty Officer Fleet/Command	MCPO
Master Chief Petty Officer of the Navy	MCPON
Master Chief Petty Officer of the Coast Guard	MCPOCG

Commissioned Officers

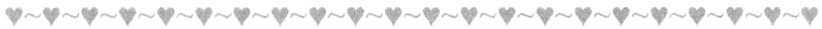

♥~♥~♥~♥~♥~♥~♥~♥~♥~♥~♥~♥~♥~♥~♥~♥~♥~♥~♥

Officers in the Army are generally addressed as 'Sir' unless there is a need to distinguish some individual (i.e. when addressing someone in a group).

If that is done, the rank and last name are used (i.e. Captain Smith). You wouldn't walk up to your boss and say, "Good morning, Colonel." Although it would be accurate, it would sound odd.

Lieutenants are an exception. Generally they are addressed as 'LT', unless the situation is formal, or the LT has a bit too high sense of self.

Air Force

O-1	Second Lieutenant	2d Lt
O-2	First Lieutenant	1st Lt
O-3	Captain	Capt
O-4	Major	Maj
O-5	Lieutenant Colonel	Lt Col
O-6	Colonel	Col
O-7	Brigadier General	Brig Gen
O-8	Major General	Maj Gen
O-9	Lieutenant General	Lt Gen
O-10	General	Gen
General of the Air Force		GAF

Army

O-1	Second Lieutenant	2LT
O-2	First Lieutenant	1LT
O-3	Captain	Cpt
O-4	Major	Maj
O-5	Lieutenant Colonel	Ltc

O-6	Colonel	Col
O-7	Brigadier General	BG
O-8	Major General	MG
O-9	Lieutenant General	LTG
O-10	General	GEN
	General of the Army	GA

Marines

O-1	Second Lieutenant	2ndLt
O-2	First Lieutenant	1stLt
O-3	Captain	Capt
O-4	Major	Maj
O-5	Lieutenant Colonel	LtCol
O-6	Colonel	Col
O-7	Brigadier General	BGen
O-8	Major General	MajGen
O-9	Lieutenant General	LtGen
O-10	General	Gen

Navy

O-1	Ensign	ENS
O-2	Lieutenant Junior Grade	LTJG
O-3	Lieutenant	Lt
O-4	Lieutenant Commander	LCDR
O-5	Commander	CDR
O-6	Captain	CAPT
O-7	Rear Admiral (Lower Half)	RDML
O-8	Rear Admiral (Upper Half)	RADM
O-9	Vice Admiral	VADM

O-10   Admiral Chief of Naval Operations/   ADM
Commandant of the CG

Fleet Admiral   FDAM

Warrant Officer Ranks

♥~♥

Warrant officer ranks are identical across the services. A 'W-1' is referred to simply as 'Warrant Officer.'

W-2 and higher are referred to as 'Chief Warrant Officer 2' or W-3 , 4 or 5 as the case may be.

Once past the rank of W-1, they are commonly addressed as 'Chief' in the Army.

A nickname for W-1's is 'spot,' referring to the single dot they have on their bar.

Royal Titles

♥~♥~♥~♥~♥~♥~♥~♥~♥~♥~♥~♥~♥~♥~♥~♥~♥~♥~♥

King~ Hereditary head of a Nation or State
Monarch   Majesty   Sovereign
Greeting: Your Royal Highness; or Sir

Queen~ Hereditary ruler
Queen Mother   Queen Dowager
Greeting: Your Royal Highness; or Madam

Prince~ The male child of a monarch. Royalty not Nobility.
Crown Prince   Prince Royal   Prince of Wales

Princess~ The female child of a Monarch. Royalty not Nobility
Princess Royal   Crown Princess

Arch Duke~ One born of Royal blood

Grand Duke~ Male title

Grand Duchess~ Female title

Duke/Duchess~ Sons or Daughters of Kings are usually given this title.
Formal Introduction: His/Her Grace, the Duke/Duchess of (*Camden/Snowden/whatever*)

Marquees/Marquis~ Male title
Formal Introduction: Lord (*Camden/Snowden/whatever*)

Marchioness/Marquise~ Female title
Formal Introduction: Lady (*Camden/Snowden/whatever*)

Earl/Count~ Male title
Formal Introduction: Lord (*Camden/Snowden/whatever*)

Countess/Contessa~ Female title
Formal Introduction: Lady (*Camden/Snowden/whatever*)

Viscount/Viscountess~ A title the king bestows on
someone who has not earned the right to be a Count; this title
is predominantly found in the UK and France.
Formal Introduction: Lord/Lady (*Camden/Snowden/area*)
Related Words~ viscountcy or viscounty

Baron/Baroness~ A large part of nobility are Barons;
those who got their lands from the King.
Formal Introduction: Lord/Lady (*Camden/Snowden/area*)
Related words~ barony, baronial, baronage

Baronet~ Hereditary Knighthood and a Noble title
Formal Introduction: Sir Simon Camden/Lady Camden (*area*)
Related Words~ baronetcy, baronetage

Knight~ A title of honor
Formal Introduction: Sir Simon (*Camden/Snowden/area*)

Five levels of British Titles~ Royalty, Nobility,
Knights, Gentry and Commons

Nobility and Peerage~ A Peer is the holder of the title
and a member of parliament.
A Noble is a member of the peer's family. The nobility are also
landowners.

Nobles and Nobility~ To be a Noble meant you were
a descendent of a diplomat or ambassador. Although the title
could be bought, it meant more to be a true Noble.

Sovereigns and Sovereignty~ To be considered
Sovereign one does not need to be royal. It is a title given to a
hereditary head of state.
To be sovereign is to be a ruling head of state, but they need not
be royal, i.e. the Pope is Sovereign.

Other Royal Titles

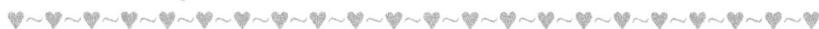

♥~♥

The Prince of Wales
The Prince of Wales is a title created for the male heir to the throne. There is no automatic succession to this title, but it is normally passed on when the existing Prince of Wales accedes to the throne.

Aide-de-Camp (ADC)
Considered an honorary appointment; the small group is appointed by the Queen.

Companion of the Queen's Service Order (QSO)
The Order was instituted by the Queen in 1975.

Duke of Cornwall/Duchy of Cornwall
One of the oldest and largest land estates in England, it provides an income for the male heir to the throne. It has been in existence for over 650 years.

Duke of Rothesay
This is the title of the Scottish peerage.

Earl of Carrick and Baron of Renfrew
A title of Scottish Peerage inherited by an heir

Earl of Chester
The position was created to keep an eye on any warlike activities of the Welsh.

Knight of the Garter (KG)
The senior British Order of Chivalry

Knight of the Thistle (KT)
The Most Ancient and Most Noble Order is Scotland's highest honor and precedes the King of the Garter.

Knight Grand Cross of the Order of the Bath (GCB)
Mainly given to officers in the armed service and sometimes a select few civil servants.

Knight of the Order of Australia (AK)
This Order was instituted by the Queen in 1975 on the advice of her Australian ministers.

Lord of The Isles
An ancient title passed to the heirs of the King of Scotland

Order of Merit (OM)
This Order is restricted to twenty-four members and is one of the most coveted titles.

Prince and Great Steward of Scotland
The title belongs to the first-born prince of the King of Scotland.

Privy Counsellor (PC)
This title includes senior ministers, leaders of opposing parties, Archbishops of both York and Canterbury. Appointment to this position is for life.

Words To Eliminate

❤~❤

The following are some of the most commonly overused:

about	all	almost
always	eagerly	every
finally	frequently	got
just	merely	nearly
need	never	not
often	only	so
that	then	very
walk		

If you've used the following words, chances are in most cases you can take them out and not miss them:

although	appeared	at least
began	even	felt
figured	for a moment	heard
if nothing else	in spite of	knew
looked	over	perhaps
quite	rather	realized
really	saw	seemed
sort of	started	suddenly
the fact that		

You can also remove - And, But or While from the beginning of a sentence

About the Author

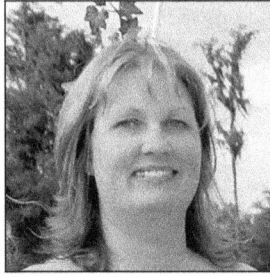

Rebecca Andrews lives in the Nevada desert with her own hero husband who makes it easy to write about the magic of romance. The mother of four grown children and grandmother to two granddaughters and a grandson, she enjoys spending her free time reading, gardening or taking in a good movie.

You can visit Rebecca at:
http://www.rebeccaandrews.net

Word of mouth is crucial for any author to succeed. If you found this book useful, please take a moment to leave a review on Amazon. Even if it's just a sentence or two, it would make all the difference and be very much appreciated.

Thanks!
Rebecca

.

www.ingramcontent.com/pod-product-compliance
Lightning Source LLC
Chambersburg PA
CBHW030004290326
41934CB00005B/223